BIRTH READY & BEYOND

YOUR HOLISTIC GUIDE FOR PREGNANCY, LABOR, & POSTPARTUM RECOVERY

BUFFY STINCHFIELD, PT

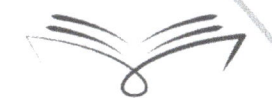

LITTLE BLACK BOOK
PUBLISHING

St Louis, MO

Copyright © 2025 Buffy Stinchfield

Little Black Book Publishing Co. All rights reserved.

No part of this publication may be reproduced, distributed, or transmitted in any form or by any means, including photocopying, recording, or other electronic or mechanical methods, without the prior written permission of the publisher, except as permitted by U.S. copyright law. For permission requests, contact Little Black Book Publishing Company at 1600 Mid Rivers Mall Dr. St Peters, MO 63376.

Published by LBB Publishing. An imprint of Little Black Book: Women in Business

Illustrations and diagrams by Cierra Biles; illustration refinement and background design by Alyssa Alarcón Santo.

Interior layout and editing by: Shelly Snow Pordea

Paperback ISBN: 978-1-962417-35-8

The Birth Ready Bundle

A companion to this book

As you move through Birth Ready & Beyond, you may find it helpful to have certain tools available in a format you can easily revisit, update, or share with your birth team.

The Birth Ready Bundle is a simple digital companion to this book. It includes printable versions of key resources referenced throughout these pages, along with trusted links many readers appreciate having in one place.

Inside the bundle, you'll find:
- birth plan checklists and a simple summary page
- partner support and hospital bag checklists
- a postpartum self-care at home checklist
- trusted resources referenced in this book

These tools are here to support your preparation in a way that feels calm and manageable—not something to complete all at once.

To access the Birth Ready Bundle, scan the QR code below and enter your email for immediate access.

This is here for you when and how you need it.

The Birth Ready Bundle is a digital resource available to readers of this book. You can unsubscribe from emails at any time.

Contents

Dedication	1
My Birth Story	2
My Prenatal and Postpartum Resource List	6
SECTION I: Healthy Foundations	8
1. The Four Pillars of Core and Pelvic Health	10
2. Understanding Your Pelvic Floor: A Vital Connection	14
3. Core & Pelvic Floor Self-Assessment	16
Breath: Connecting to Your Core and Pelvic Floor	
Alignment: Wall Lean Exercise	
Coordination: The Core and Pelvic Floor	
Hip Strength: The Hip Hinge Challenge	
4. Pelvic Floor Screening and Self-Assessment	25
Pelvic Floor Screening	
5. Your Core and Breathing	34
6. Focus for Labor Preparation	42
7. Health Tips While Pregnant	48
8. Nutrition Essentials During Pregnancy and Postpartum	54
9. Prenatal Exercises	64

10.	Self-Care Challenge By Trimester	76
	Self-Care Assessments, Goals, & Self-Care Bingos	

SECTION II: Preparing to Push — 91

11.	How am I Supposed to Prepare to Push?	93
12.	Timeline for Birth Preparation	96
13.	The Best Labor Positions	100
14.	The Glottis, Jaw, And The Pelvic Floor	104
15.	By 30 Weeks; Inversions and Being on All Fours	106
16.	Preventing Perineal Tears	108
17.	Birth Coaching with Pelvic PTs/OTs	114
18.	Back and Belly Support	118
	Taping vs Bracing	
19.	Recommended Actions Steps: Third Trimester Through Birth	120

Reflection Journal Pages — 124

SECTION III: Labor Support — 127

20.	Your Birth Environment	128
21.	Guiding Each Labor Stage: Goals and Partner Support	132
	Stage 1: Early Labor	
	Transition	
	Stage 2: Pushing Stage	

Partner Support Checklist — 141

22.	Labor Support Tools and Techniques	143
23.	The Best Birthing Positions For The Pushing Phase	154

Illustrated Birthing Positions	155
24. Jaw, Neck, and Shoulder Tension Relieving Strategies Before and During Birth	157
25. Vocalization Channeling Strength and Releasing Tension in Labor	160
26. Using Inflatable Devices:	164
Illustrated Birth Positions with CUB	166
Illustrated Birth Positions with Peanut Ball	169
29. When Is it Time to Push?	171
30. Mindset and Affirmations	174
31. Crafting Your Birth Plan	184
32. What to Pack in Your Hospital (or Birth Center) Bag	190
33. Preparing for Labor: Foods and Teas to Consider in the Final 4-6 Weeks	195
SECTION IV: Postpartum Recovery	202
34. 5-5-5 Rule	206
35. Supporting Your Recovery: Signs to Watch, Self-Care, and When to Seek Medical Care	210
36. Postpartum Recovery in Weeks 0-6 The Core Four	219
37. Postpartum Nutrition	224
38. Favorite Postpartum Recipes	229

39. Lactation Support	235
Breastfeeding Recommendations from the World Health Organization (WHO)	
40. Early Core Restoration	238
New Mom Stretches	243
41. When to See a Pelvic Physical or Occupational Therapist Postpartum	246
42. Your Next Steps	254
Healing, Thriving, and Beyond	
43. Your Birth Story	260
Reflect and Cherish	
Birth Ready Resources	266
About the Author	270

Dedication

To my mother, Teresa Dettman,
Your unwavering love and belief in me have shaped everything I do.

In 2019, you called to share a vivid dream you had about me writing a book—a dream so real you said it felt as though you were holding the finished pages in your hands. At the time, I hadn't told anyone about my quiet intention to write this book, yet you saw it before I could.

When you passed in 2022, the grief was heavy, but your dream stayed with me. It became my guiding light, reminding me that this work wasn't just about me—it was about fulfilling a purpose larger than myself.

This book is for the women you believed I could help, and for you, Mom. Your vision gave me the courage to see it through. I miss you every day, but your dream lives on in these pages.

With all my love,
Buffy

My Birth Story

In the midst of shock and pain, I found myself dragging my nine-months pregnant body across the hospital floor where I worked. I had slipped, falling onto the wet pool room floor where I'd just finished working with a patient, only days before my planned maternity leave. The absurdity of my situation left me laughing through my tears.

As my colleagues rushed to my aid, I was certain my lower right leg was broken. In this case, working near an orthopedic department was a small silver lining. Wheeled into the surgeon's office, Panic set in; the natural birth I had envisioned seemed impossible. This moment marked the beginning of a journey I never anticipated.

The following days were filled with uncertainty. In the OB-GYN's office, I expected to undergo an immediate induction or C-section. Instead, the doctor calmly suggested we wait another week for labor to start naturally. I felt dismissed and invalidated, enduring the cumulative physical toll of the broken leg, sciatica, swelling, and pelvic pain. Each day felt like an eternity, an expansive mix of hope and frustration.

Two weeks later, still pregnant and using crutches, I was back at the hospital to be induced. Determined to be the "good" patient, I accepted that I would be laboring with a broken leg. When the nurse prompted me to start pushing, I didn't stop to check in with my own body—I pushed on command, for three exhausting hours. When my baby boy finally arrived, the joy of his birth was marred by exhaustion and the overwhelming feeling of being utterly broken.

Looking back, I can see all the ways my birth experience was shaped by a lack of preparation and guidance. My broken leg complicated things, but it was my lack of understanding about the birth process (despite taking the hospital birth class), poor mental and physical preparation, and inadequate resources that made things much harder than they needed to be. I had completely outsourced my birth experience to others—most of whom I had never met before. I don't wish that for anyone else.

Right after my son was born, it took an hour for my doctor to stitch my pelvic floor, and later, when I tried to hop to the bathroom on crutches, my bladder control failed. I felt like the poster child for birth trauma.

In those early postpartum days, self-care felt like an impossible luxury. The mainstream approach seemed focused solely on weight gain or loss during pregnancy, leaving me woefully unprepared for the reality of birth recovery. I assumed my body would just bounce back on its own, as so many of us are led to believe. I desperately needed pelvic physical therapy in those early weeks and months—but I didn't know it existed, and my doctor never mentioned it.

Around five or six months postpartum, I finally began to feel physically stronger. I was fortunate and my desire to specialize in pelvic physical therapy was born to help myself heal fully. But even more than that, it was a turning point; one that sparked my desire to help other women reclaim their strength and confidence after pregnancy.

Beyond Kegels: Bridging the Gap in Birth Preparation

After a few years as a pelvic physical therapist, I began to see the gaps in how women were being prepared for childbirth. Most prenatal care focuses on the baby's health and safety, leaving the mother's physical and emotional needs unaddressed. The reality is that most of us are not taught how to connect with our breath, core, or our pelvic floor. We are also rarely taught how to feel mentally prepared for childbirth. The difference these tools can make is incredible.

Since 2012, I've helped my patients prepare their bodies and minds for childbirth. Together, we focus on enhancing pelvic and hip mobility, coordinating breath with pelvic floor movements, and exploring optimal birthing positions. It's not just about physical preparation—it's about mental readiness, emotional resilience, and empowering women to feel confident in their choices.

A Call to Action

This book is the resource I wish I had before my first birth. It's designed to support you holistically—physically, mentally, and nutritionally—as you navigate pregnancy, childbirth, and postpartum recovery. Whether this is your first baby or an opportunity to create a more empowered experience after a previous birth, my hope is that these pages will equip you with the tools, guidance, and encouragement you need to approach this transformative time with strength and confidence.

Let this book be your companion on this journey. You deserve to feel prepared, supported, and empowered every step of the way.

Disclaimer:

The information provided in this book is intended for general informational purposes only and is not a substitute for professional medical advice, diagnosis, or treatment. Always seek the advice of your physician or other qualified health provider with any questions you may have regarding a medical condition.

The content in this book is based on general knowledge and practices and may not be suitable for every individual. Consult with your healthcare provider before making any significant changes to your exercise, nutrition, or lifestyle, especially if you are pregnant or planning to become pregnant.

The author and publisher of this book are not responsible for any specific health or medical needs that may require medical supervision and are not liable for any damages or negative consequences from any treatment, action, application, or preparation, to any person reading or following the information in this book.

My Prenatal and Postpartum Resource List

Finding these resources in your town now, will help you prepare for and build your personal care team to have now and in your postpartum journey.

Birth Provider:

- *Name:*

- *Email/phone*

Birth Location:

- *Name:*

- *Website/phone:*

Pelvic Physical Therapist/ Occupational Therapist

- *Name:*

- *Email/phone*

Prenatal/Postpartum Chiropractor:

- *Name:*

- *Email/phone:*

Doula:

- *Name:*

- *Email/phone:*

Lactation Counselor/Consultant:

- *Name:*

- *Email/phone:*

Your Birth Space: Hospital, Birth Center, or Home

Where you choose to give birth is a personal decision shaped by your values, your medical needs, and the care options available to you. Whether you're planning a hospital birth, a birth center experience, or a home birth, the principles in this book are here to support you through a vaginal birth in any setting. Even though I include tools like a hospital packing list, everything in these pages is meant to help you feel prepared, grounded, and confident—wherever you welcome your baby. Over the years, I've supported women across all settings, and I've seen how preparation, mindset, and body awareness can create meaningful and empowering birth experiences in each one.

SECTION I: Healthy Foundations

When it comes to being pregnant, it is easy to jump ahead mentally and focus on the birth, your new baby, and all the other fun details of this exciting time. I can remember spending many hours searching for names, studying how large my baby was that week, and what I wanted their room to be decorated like.

Wherever you are in your pregnancy journey, *now* is the time to focus on establishing or maintaining healthy foundations for your body. We all have things that we are better at with self care than others, so now is the time to begin to refocus on where you are, and where you want to be.

When it comes to physically preparing your body for labor, it is important to understand that birth involves the connection of both the mind and body. We cannot mentally disconnect from our body and hope for our birth experience to be an ideal physiologic vaginal birth. So as we move forward in helping you prepare for your birth, realize that your prenatal exercises and breath work is intentionally a mind-body practice.

Let's begin by focusing on core and pelvic health foundations. Following this, we will proceed with a guided self-assessment.

This section covers *Healthy Foundations*:

- 4 Pillars of Core & Pelvic Health: The KEY to a healthy pregnancy, delivery and recovery

- Understanding Your Pelvic Floor: A Vital Connection

- Core and Pelvic Health Self Assessment

- Cozean Pelvic Health Quiz and Pelvic Health Home Self-Assessment

- Your Core and Breathing

- Focus for Labor Prep

- Physical Goals While Pregnant

- Health Tips While Pregnant

- Key Nutrients Recommended During Pregnancy and Postpartum

- Core Prenatal Exercises

- Homework Time!

- Self Care Assessment, Goal Setting, and Self Care Challenge By Trimester

- Journal Pages for Healthy Foundations

Chapter 1
The Four Pillars of Core and Pelvic Health

THE DEEP CORE AND pelvic floor muscles have common basic needs regardless of the person or issue. Over the years practicing as a pelvic physical therapist, I have found that there are 4 main pillars of pelvic floor and core health that we all need regardless of the issue or phase of life. While pregnant, thinking in terms of these 4 pillars will help you now during your pregnancy, during labor and in your postpartum recovery journey.

1. **Breath:** Breath is the foundation of core and pelvic floor muscle function. Through healthy and coordinated breath, our core muscle health can be restored and or maintained. In the journey to restore core and pelvic floor health, breath will always be a part of the first steps. While pregnant, breath work will help you to prepare to use your breath as a powerhouse tool during your labor too!

2. **Alignment:** Our muscles can only work optimally when our bodies are aligned well. Poor body positioning can put muscles into excessively long or short positions which can make them extra tense or not be able to turn on at all. Additionally, imbalances in hip, back and pelvic muscles can contribute to unwanted preg-

nancy aches and pains in the back and pelvis.

3. **Coordination, then Strength of the Core and Pelvic Floor Muscles:** Our deep core muscles need to first be able to coordinate together as a *team* before we can focus on getting stronger. This includes when pelvic floor muscles are stuck in a short tense position. We must first help them to regain normal tension/length before it is appropriate to improve strength. Repetitively tensing pelvic floor muscles alone, will only lead to more leakage, pain, or pressure issues. When we are preparing for birth, the *last* thing we need is pelvic floor muscles that are unable to let go! The focus here will be on finding how to best *release* your pelvic floor in multiple positions.

4. **Hip Strength:** Our hip/glute muscles are the foundation for our back, hip, knee, core, and pelvic health. Poorly activating glutes are an epidemic in chair using societies (non squatting societies). Regaining the ability to fully access our glute muscles can help resolve back pain, hip flexor tension, pelvic floor dysfunction, and core weakness. Pelvic floor muscles cannot function well if the glutes cannot stabilize and move the pelvis effectively. Through the course of our pregnancies, women are often shocked to realize that their glutes become weak along with their abdominals by the time they deliver their baby. While we cannot prevent some loss of strength of the core and glutes, we can certainly work to maintain and even increase our glute strength throughout our pregnancy.

Start with your foundation, and everything else will follow.

Chapter 2
Understanding Your Pelvic Floor: A Vital Connection

MANY WOMEN HAVE BEEN told to "do Kegels" or "engage their core" in fitness classes or by well-meaning providers. However, the concept of connecting these muscles to their breath and, just as importantly, learning to relax them on purpose as a skill is rarely emphasized—yet it's a crucial foundation for pelvic health and birth preparation. Perhaps they've experienced the occasional bladder leak, a moment of discomfort during intimacy, or even no issues at all. Yet, when it comes to labor and birth, this often-overlooked area of the body takes center stage. Surprisingly, a majority of the women I treat—more than 75%—have an excess of pelvic floor tension. And while these muscles are vital, the ability to consciously release that tension on command is a skill that most have never been taught.

Labor is not the ideal time to learn this skill for the first time. In the midst of contractions and the demands of birth, our thinking brain often steps aside, leaving us reliant on instincts and preparation. Hoping that a nurse, doula, or birth provider will intuitively offer the exact words or cues to help release pelvic floor tension is a gamble that no birthing woman should have to take. That's why learning to connect with and release your pelvic floor muscles in a safe, calm environment—whether at home or in the care of a pelvic health provider—is so critical. Even without an internal muscle assessment, we can explore these connections through verbal guidance, gentle tactile cues, and supportive positions. Every woman deserves this opportunity.

This is why I've included a pelvic floor self-assessment in this book. Not everyone has access to a pelvic health therapist, feels comfortable seeking one, or knows where to start. This simple assessment is designed to empower you with knowledge of your anatomy, help you determine whether you can connect with your pelvic floor muscles, and identify any tenderness or tension. For some, this may be the first time truly reflecting on this part of the body. If you find concerns during your self-assessment, know that there are pelvic health therapists dedicated to guiding women out of shame, pain, and dysfunction toward thriving in every aspect of life. My hope is that this assessment will serve as a gateway to greater awareness, empowerment, and, ultimately, confidence as you prepare for birth and beyond.

Chapter 3
Core & Pelvic Floor Self-Assessment

THIS SELF-ASSESSMENT IS DESIGNED to help you gain insight into your core and pelvic health—similar to the screenings I regularly conduct with in-person clients. It uses simple tools you likely already have at home and will give you a practical, foundational understanding of where you currently stand.

Combined with the **Cozean Pelvic Health Screen**, this assessment can provide valuable insights to share with a pelvic health physical therapist (PT), occupational therapist (OT), or your birth provider. Whether you identify areas of concern or simply want to understand your body better, this information can be a powerful step toward feeling more prepared and confident.

What You'll Need:

- A balloon

- A dowel, broom, or yardstick (at least 3 feet long)

Breath: Connecting to Your Core and Pelvic Floor

Breath Awareness Exercise:

1. Begin in a seated position with your feet on the floor and your back supported, or sit cross-legged with your back supported.

2. Place one hand on your chest and the other on your belly.

3. Slowly take a 4-count *inhale* through your nose, allowing the air to fill your lungs.

4. Exhale slowly for 4 counts through pursed lips, focusing on a controlled release.

5. Repeat this process 2–3 times.

Q: Where did most of the movement occur—your chest, your belly, or equally in both? Use the space below to record your observation:

Finding Your Belly Breath: Now, aim to direct most of the movement into your belly, allowing it to gently expand downward toward your pelvic floor as you inhale.

Q: Was it easy or difficult to shift the movement lower into your belly? Write down your thoughts:

Exploring Different Postures: Try practicing this belly breathing exercise in the following postures to see how each feels. The goal is to find a position where your belly can expand and relax with ease. (Note: When facing downward, allow your belly to naturally release toward the floor with each inhale.)

- **Laying on your side:** Tip your top shoulder slightly back for added comfort.

- **Hands and knees:** Keep your hips over your knees and let your belly hang gently.

- **Child's Pose:** Sit back onto your heels, arms extended forward, and let your belly rest toward your thighs.

- **Sitting while leaning forward:** Rest your arms on a table or surface for support.

Q: Which posture felt easiest for allowing your belly to relax and expand naturally? Reflect and record your answer:

Why This Matters: Your breath is a powerful tool for calming your nervous system, connecting with your pelvic floor, and preparing for labor. By practicing in different postures, you'll discover which position allows you to let go of tension most effectively—this can be especially helpful during labor or moments of stress.

Alignment: Wall Lean Exercise

Wall Lean Setup:

1. Stand with your feet about 18 inches away from a wall.

2. Allow your knees to remain softly bent.

3. Align your entire back, including your head, so it rests gently against the wall.

4. Place your hands on your belly to connect with your breathing. **Bonus:** Take 3 slow belly breaths in this position.

Q: Were you able to align your head and back along the wall with ease, or did you find it challenging? Use the space below to jot down your observations:

Why This Matters: This wall lean exercise serves as both a check-in for your posture and a tool for alignment as your belly grows and your body adjusts. By periodically practicing this position, you'll develop a better sense of what "neutral alignment" feels like.

If you find it challenging to engage your core muscles during your day, the wall lean can help you reconnect. Try this:

- As you exhale or blow out through pursed lips, gently draw your belly back toward the wall, engaging your core muscles. This action will help your back press closer to the wall.

Added Benefits: After practicing the wall lean, you can enhance flexibility and stretch your back:

- Press your low back gently into the wall.

- Reach your arms and shoulders forward, creating space in your back.

- Take a few deep breaths, focusing on expanding your upper or lower back as you inhale. This stretch promotes lengthening and relaxation in the back muscles.

Coordination: The Core and Pelvic Floor

This part of the assessment helps you understand how well your core and pelvic floor muscles coordinate during common tasks like blowing or coughing. Let's check in with two simple exercises.

Option 1: The Balloon Challenge

- Sit tall with your feet on the floor and your back supported.

- Take a nice, full inhale to prepare.

- Exhale with one strong effort to blow into a balloon.

- Pay attention to the following:

    - Did your belly move inward or bulge outward?

    - Did you feel any pressure pushing downward onto your pelvic floor?

Q: How did your core and pelvic floor respond?

Option 2: The Cough Test

- Sit in a slightly reclined position with your feet on the floor.

- Place one hand on your belly.

- Do a single, strong cough and notice what happens:

    - Did your belly move inward or outward?

    - Did your pelvic floor lift or push downward?

Q: What did you observe during the cough?

What These Tests Reveal: Ideally, your core and pelvic floor muscles should coordinate with the diaphragm as it moves. In both the balloon blow and the cough, a well-coordinated core team will draw the belly and pelvic floor inward and upward as the diaphragm moves upward during exhalation.

If you notice a lack of coordination or feel downward pressure on your pelvic floor, this is valuable information to share with a pelvic health PT or OT for further guidance.

Hip Strength: The Hip Hinge Challenge

Mastering the hip hinge is key to strengthening your glutes and protecting your back. Strong, engaged glutes support your pelvis, back, and overall movement, making this exercise an essential foundation for pregnancy, postpartum, and beyond.

What You'll Need: A dowel, broom, yardstick, or similar object.

How to Perform the Hip Hinge Challenge:

1. **Set Up:**

   - Stand tall with your feet about hip-width apart.

   - Place the dowel along your back so it touches three key points:

     - The back of your head.

     - Your mid-back (around the bra line).

     - Your tailbone.

2. **Engage Your Glutes:**

   - Before moving, gently rotate your thigh bones outward. This outward rotation activates your glutes while keeping your tailbone untucked.

   - Avoid clenching or squeezing too tightly—focus on a subtle, controlled engagement.

3. **Hinge at Your Hips:**

   - Picture yourself bowing politely to someone. This movement starts by hinging your hips backward rather than moving your body downward.

   - Keep the dowel in contact with all three points (head, mid-back, and tailbone) as you hinge.

- Maintain the natural curve of your lower back throughout the movement. If your lower back begins to flatten or align with the dowel, your low back muscles are likely taking over, and your glutes are disengaged. Stop immediately and return to the starting position.

- Stop hinging at around a 40–45 degree angle. There's no need to hinge further or bring your body parallel to the floor—quality of movement is the goal, not depth.

What to Observe:

- Can you maintain contact with all three points on the dowel during the hinge?

- Were you able to keep your lower back's natural curve intact, or did it flatten against the dowel?

- Are your glutes staying active throughout the motion, or do they "turn off" partway through?

Q: Were you able to keep the dowel in contact with all three points?

Q: How far were you able to hinge while keeping your glutes activated and maintaining the natural curve of your lower back?

Why This Matters: The hip hinge is an essential movement pattern for everyday life—whether you're picking up toys, lifting your baby, or performing daily tasks. Many people mistakenly bend from their lower back or knees, leading to overuse and potential injury. By focusing on hinging your hips backward and activating your glutes, you'll build strength, reduce strain on your knees and back, and create better overall movement habits.

This test may sound simple, but it's surprisingly difficult for most people. In the 12 years since I created this test with patients, 90% struggle to hinge properly without relying on their lower back muscles. Practicing this movement regularly will improve your coordination and strength over time.

Pro Tip: If you notice your lower back begins to tense or flatten against the dowel, stop the hinge and return to the starting position. Try to reset and focus on engaging your glutes properly, and hinge only to the point you can feel your glutes (and not low back muscles) on. The goal is quality over depth—stop at a 40–45 degree angle to maintain alignment.

Remember, this is just a screen. If you find this movement challenging, don't be discouraged! I have many other ways to help patients retrain their hip hinge that don't look like this test or feel as potentially frustrating.

Chapter 4
Pelvic Floor Screening and Self-Assessment

The Cozean Screening Protocol was designed as a simple yet effective tool to help individuals and their healthcare providers identify potential pelvic floor dysfunction. Completing this quick screening can provide valuable insights into your pelvic health. If your score is 3 or higher, it strongly indicates the likelihood of pelvic floor dysfunction, and you would greatly benefit from an evaluation with a pelvic health physical therapist.

Pelvic Floor Screening

Instructions: *Check all that apply to you. Please answer each question by selecting* **Yes** *or* **No**.

1. Pelvic Pain

I sometimes or occasionally have pelvic pain (in the genitals, perineum, pubic area, or bladder area), or pain with urination, that exceeds a **3** on a **1–10 pain scale** (with 10 being the worst pain imaginable).

☐ Yes   ☐ No

2. History of Falls or Trauma

I can remember falling onto my **tailbone, lower back, or buttocks** (even during childhood).

☐ Yes   ☐ No

3. Urinary Symptoms

I sometimes experience **one or more** of the following urinary symptoms:

- Accidental loss of urine (incontinence)
- Feeling unable to completely empty my bladder
- Needing to urinate again within a few minutes of a previous void
- Pain or burning with urination
- Difficulty starting, stopping, or maintaining a steady urine stream

☐ Yes   ☐ No

4. Nighttime Urination

I sometimes or occasionally have to get up to urinate **two or more times per night**.

☐ Yes   ☐ No

5. Pelvic Pressure

I sometimes have the feeling of **increased pelvic pressure** or the sensation that my pelvic organs are **slipping down or falling out**.

☐ Yes   ☐ No

6. Musculoskeletal Pain History

I have a history of pain in my **low back, hips, groin, or tailbone**, or I have experienced **sciatica**.

☐ Yes ☐ No

7. Bowel Symptoms

I sometimes experience **one or more** of the following bowel symptoms:

- Loss of bowel control
- Feeling unable to completely empty my bowels
- Straining or pain with bowel movements
- Difficulty initiating a bowel movement

☐ Yes ☐ No

8. Pain With Sexual Activity

I sometimes experience **pain or discomfort with sexual activity or intercourse**.

☐ Yes ☐ No

9. Symptom Flare After Sexual Activity

I notice that sexual activity **increases one or more of my other symptoms**.

☐ Yes ☐ No

10. Sitting Intolerance

Prolonged sitting increases my symptoms.

☐ Yes   ☐ No

If you checked *yes* to three or more questions, pelvic floor dysfunction is likely. You may benefit from an assessment by a pelvic floor physical therapist.

The Cozean Pelvic Health Screen was developed by Jesse and Nicole Cozean at Pelvic Sanity

Pelvic Floor Home Self-Assessment

Many women have never taken a mirror to look at their own vulvar anatomy. This is common and often stems from disconnection or discomfort around this part of the body. It's understandable, especially if you've experienced pelvic pain, incontinence, painful periods, a history of trauma or abuse, or come from a culture that reinforces body shaming. If this resonates with you, know that you're not alone, and exploring this part of yourself is an important step toward reclaiming your connection to your body.

This home self-assessment is designed to be a starting point for you to reconnect with your pelvic floor in the privacy and comfort of your own space. It's about curiosity and learning what is your "normal" before you go through your upcoming birth. This self-assessment does not replace a comprehensive evaluation by a trauma-informed, skilled pelvic floor physical therapist. However, it can provide valuable insight into your pelvic health and serve as a foundation for discussions with a pelvic PT.

If you have a history of pelvic issues or discover something new during this assessment, connecting with a pelvic therapist can be an empowering step in your pregnancy journey. They can help you deepen your awareness, release tension, and support your body through this significant transition.

Using a Pelvic Wand for Self-Assessment

A pelvic wand is a specially designed tool that allows women to assess and address the muscles of their pelvic floor. The **Intimate Rose Pelvic Wand** is a popular choice due to its ergonomic design and ease of use. Made with velvety soft, medical-grade silicone, the original purple wand is shaped to reach all areas of the pelvic floor with comfort and precision.

During pregnancy, many women find it increasingly difficult to evaluate their own pelvic floor muscles as their body changes. The pelvic wand offers a solution by making it easier to reach and assess for areas of muscle tension or tenderness. Postpartum, the wand can be an invaluable tool for evaluating the pelvic floor as it heals, helping you locate any discomfort or tightness that may need attention.

This gentle assessment can also serve as an important first step before deciding when you might feel ready to be intimate with your partner again. By identifying and addressing areas of tension or tenderness, the pelvic wand supports your journey toward regaining comfort and confidence in your body.

If you're unsure about using a pelvic wand or how it fits into your recovery, be sure to consult a pelvic health physical therapist for guidance tailored to your needs.

Steps to Perform Your Home Self-Assessment

1. Get into a comfortable, supported position: Recline with your back supported and your knees bent and relaxed. Use pillows or cushions for support as needed.

2. Visualize your anatomy: Take a mirror and gently observe your vulva and vaginal opening. This step helps you become familiar with your own anatomy and establishes a baseline for what feels and looks normal for you.

3. Use a finger/thumb or pelvic wand with lubricant: Lightly apply lubricant to your finger or pelvic wand. Insert it about 1 inch into your vaginal opening, and gently press down towards your tailbone and to each side. Be mindful of how this feels and note any points of tenderness or discomfort.

4. Assess your response to gentle pressure and breath: If you find a tender spot, maintain very light pressure over it and take three slow, deep breaths. Does the tenderness decrease? A gentle release of tension in response to your breath can be a good sign of your body's ability to let go.

Next Steps

If you discover tender spots or significant tension, it's recommended that you seek out a pelvic therapist. They can help you connect your breath to your pelvic floor and teach you techniques to release tension.

If you don't notice tenderness but sense some tension, you can gently massage the lower half of your perineum using a finger, thumb, or pelvic wand. This massage can help you prepare for your delivery by increasing your awareness and reducing muscle tightness in the perineal area.

By exploring this part of your body, you're taking a proactive step toward supporting yourself during pregnancy and birth. Remember, this is about getting curious and understanding your body—not achieving perfection. If at any point you feel unsure or have concerns, reach out to a trauma-informed pelvic PT for personalized care and guidance.

After completing the Cozean Pelvic Health Screen and pelvic floor self-assessment, you have a better understanding of your body's core and pelvic health. Next, we'll delve into breathing techniques, followed by prenatal exercises and nutrition education for a healthy mom and baby. You may share any of the self-tests in this book with your pelvic therapist or birth provider to receive more support during your journey.

Notes:

Awareness is the first step to healing. Take this moment to connect with your body and understand its unique needs.

Chapter 5
Your Core and Breathing

Breathing is more than just taking in oxygen—it's a vital link between your core muscles and pelvic floor. Learning how to coordinate your breath with these muscles can improve strength, balance, and relaxation throughout pregnancy and beyond. This foundational practice supports proper muscle coordination, lowers stress, and enhances your ability to engage your core effectively during labor, delivery, and recovery. Let's begin with a closer look at how your core and breath work together to support your body.

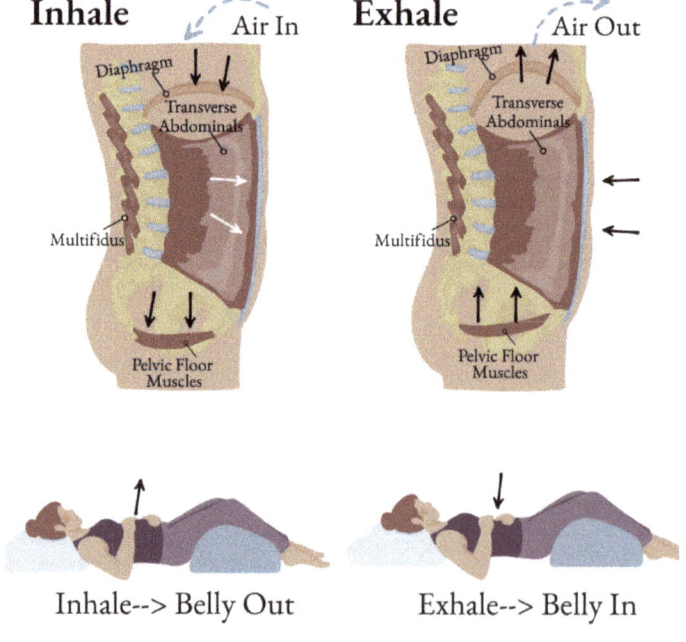

A Deeper Look

How Can This Help?

Diaphragmatic breathing, or belly breathing, is a technique that plays a critical role in pelvic floor health. When practiced regularly, it helps establish proper coordination between the diaphragm and the pelvic floor muscles, which work in sync to support movement and relaxation. This practice can:

- Improve blood flow and oxygen delivery.

- Lower stress, heart rate, and blood pressure.

- Enhance muscle function and coordination.

Mechanics of Belly Breathing

- **Inhale:** As you breathe in, the diaphragm moves downward, creating more space for the air in your lungs. This movement causes your belly to rise while the pelvic floor relaxes and stretches downward.

- **Exhale:** As you breathe out, the diaphragm moves upward to expel air, and the pelvic floor gently contracts to provide support. The belly naturally falls inward.

Visualization Technique

Imagine a balloon inside your belly:

- As you breathe in, the balloon inflates, expanding in all directions, while your pelvic floor relaxes and lengthens.

- As you breathe out, the balloon deflates, your belly contracts, and your pelvic floor gently recoils upward.

Steps to Practice Belly Breathing

1. Lie on your back with your knees bent or supported by pillows, or sit in a comfortable reclined position.

2. Rest one hand lightly on your stomach and the other on your chest.

3. Inhale gently through your nose for a count of 4, letting your stomach rise as the pelvic floor lengthens and relaxes..

4. Exhale softly through pursed lips for a slow count of 6-10, allowing your stomach to fall as the pelvic floor contracts.

5. Practice steady, intentional breathing for 3–5 minutes daily to build this connection.

Breathwork: Your Key to a Relaxed and Empowered Labor

One of the most powerful tools you can bring to your birth experience is diaphragmatic, or belly, breathing. This simple yet profound practice helps your nervous system shift into a parasympathetic state—often called the "rest and digest" mode. When your brain receives signals that you're safe and calm, it keeps the fight-or-flight response at bay, which is crucial for a stress-free, relaxed labor. Think of it as telling your body, "All is well—there's no lion chasing me!"

Breathing isn't just about oxygen—it's a direct input to your nervous system, making it one of the most effective ways to reduce your perception of pain and create an optimal environment for labor. Enhancing this practice with sensory inputs can deepen its calming effects. Consider the following:

- **Soothing smells:** Incorporate pure therapeutic grade essential oils like lavender or citrus into your breathing routine. A favorite among my patients is Balance by DoTerra, a grounding blend that complements deep, rhythmic breathing. Apply 1-2 drops to a cotton ball for easy removal if the scent feels overwhelming.

- **Music:** Relaxing tracks or meditative binaural beats can create an atmosphere of calm, encouraging a slower, more intentional breath pattern.

- **Gentle touch:** Massage or calming pressure from your birth partner can help you stay connected to your body as you breathe.

- **Dim lighting:** Battery-powered tea lights, candles or soft lamps can transform your environment into a soothing space, reducing external stressors as you focus inward.

When paired with breathwork, these sensory inputs provide a powerful way to regulate your nervous system and enhance relaxation throughout labor.

Make Breathwork a Daily Habit

If you do nothing else to prepare for birth, establishing a daily breathing practice should be a top priority. Just 3-5 minutes a day can make a significant difference in how your body and mind respond to labor.

Start by finding a posture that feels relaxing and allows you to comfortably breathe into your belly:

- Reclined with pillows supporting your back.

- On your side with your top shoulder tipped slightly back (avoid curling into a fetal posture, as it can signal fight-or-flight to your body).

- Child's Pose with your hips back and arms extended forward.

- Sitting while leaning over a bed or surface with pillows propped under your chest and arms.

As you practice, combine your breathwork with the sensory tools that resonate most with you. For example, practice belly breathing while diffusing your favorite essential oil or listening to calming music. Over time, these sensory connections will deepen, becoming second nature during labor.

Habit Stacking: Weaving Breathwork Into Your Day

Breathwork can also be your gateway to mindfulness. Even if you've never practiced mindfulness before, your breath provides a natural anchor to bring you into the present moment. The beauty of this practice is that it doesn't require a dedicated 20 minutes—it can fit seamlessly into the moments you already have.

- Take one slow, deep belly breath every time you park your car before walking into work or errands.

- Use the start of your workday as a cue—before you dive into emails, sit at your desk, and take three intentional breaths.

- When waiting in line at the grocery store or picking up your child, silently focus on extending your exhales to calm your nervous system.

- Set a timer for five minutes after you lie down in bed at night. If you fall asleep, that's okay—your body is still benefiting from the few intentional breaths you took.

Habit stacking makes it easier to stay consistent, and over time, these small moments of connection will become second nature, helping you stay calm and centered even during labor.

Tips for Building Consistency

- **Choose a Time That Works for You:** Before bed, upon waking, or during a midday pause—whatever fits best into your routine.

- **Use a Timer:** Set a timer on your phone so you don't need to watch the clock. This allows you to focus fully on your breathing.

- **Focus on Your Breath:**

  - **Inhale:** Breathe in through your nose for a count of 4, releasing tension as you expand your belly and pelvic floor, like a balloon inflating. Pause for a moment at the top of your breath.

  - **Exhale:** Softly blow out through pursed lips for a slow count of 6-10, allowing your belly and pelvic floor to deflate and naturally recoil. Take your time to avoid letting all your air out in one burst.

Journal Prompt:

Reflect on your breath work practice to deepen your connection and track your progress:

- What is the best time of day to work on my breathing?

- Which posture(s) do I feel I can belly breathe in most effectively?

- How does belly breathing feel to me? Is it calming, challenging, or both?

My breath is my body's anchor—steady, calm, and powerful.

Chapter 6
Focus for Labor Preparation

Preparing for labor is about more than just your physical readiness; it's about creating a balance between strength, relaxation, and adaptability. These are the main areas I hope every patient grasps as they prepare for their due date. In my hour-long birth coaching sessions, there's never enough time to cover everything in one sitting—I often share bits and pieces of these concepts over multiple visits. Seeing the big picture can feel overwhelming at first, but it's also incredibly calming to know there's a clear roadmap to guide you. Remember, this is a journey, and every small step adds up to a more confident, empowered birth experience.

1. Release Tension in Your Pelvic Floor and Hips

Your pelvic floor and hip muscles play a critical role in childbirth. They need to release tension and lengthen to allow your baby to pass through the pelvis. This is why the traditional advice of doing repetitive Kegels isn't always appropriate for expecting mothers. While strong pelvic floor muscles are important, muscles that remain locked in tension can lead to prolonged labor, perineal tearing, or the need for interventions such as forceps, vacuum, or episiotomy.

Most of the pelvic health patients I've worked with since 2010 have had issues rooted in excessive pelvic floor tension and difficulty relaxing on command. Identifying and addressing these issues during pregnancy can make a significant difference in labor. Pelvic health physical therapists are uniquely trained to help you recognize and release this tension, making labor smoother and reducing the risk of complications.

2. Connect Your Breath to Your Core

Your breath is a powerful tool for labor. Learning to connect diaphragmatic (belly) breathing to your core muscles—including your abdominals and pelvic floor—allows you to achieve optimal relaxation during the first stage of labor and effective pushing during the second stage. This connection not only reduces tension but also supports your body in working as a coordinated system during labor.

3. Understand and Connect with Your Pelvic Floor

For many women, the pelvic floor is an unfamiliar part of their body. Before labor, it's helpful to develop a connection with these muscles and learn to contract and release them intentionally. This awareness can reduce fear and improve your ability to work with your body during labor.If you haven't done so yet, revisit the Pelvic Health Home Self-Assessment section. This guided exercise will help you understand your pelvic floor's "normal" state and establish a deeper connection before birth.

4. Practice Different Birth Postures

Hollywood often depicts women giving birth lying on their backs with legs in stirrups, but this position is rarely optimal for the mother or baby. It limits movement of the tailbone, narrows the pelvic outlet, and offers no gravity assistance. Instead, focus on practicing positions that are more supportive for labor and delivery, including:

- Hands and knees.

- Supported hands and knees (with props like a CUB).

- Side-lying with the top leg supported by a peanut ball or cushion.

- Upright or slightly reclined sitting (such as on a birthing stool).

Begin by practicing belly breathing in each of these positions. Can you fully relax your pelvic floor, hips, and belly? Do certain positions feel more natural or effective for you? Exploring these postures ahead of time will help you feel more confident and comfortable during labor.

5. Build Core, Hip, and Shoulder Strength

Labor and motherhood are physically demanding, and strength training is crucial for meeting these challenges. Strong core and glute muscles can help you squat, bend, and lift with ease—essential tasks for caring for a baby. Similarly, shoulder strength is vital for supporting your upper body during hands-and-knees labor postures, one of the most recommended positions for delivery.

Incorporating weight-bearing exercises like push-ups, planks, squats or resistance training into your prenatal routine will not only prepare you for labor but also prevent common postpartum issues like back pain. For extra support, the "CUB" birth prop can be a game changer, especially for maintaining a supported hands-and-knees position during labor.

6. Cultivate a Calm and Flexible Mindset

Your mindset plays a powerful role in how you experience labor. To make surges (contractions) more manageable, practice achieving a state of calm by focusing on your breath and listening to your body. This helps reduce the intensity of the experience and keeps you grounded.

At the same time, it's important to balance preparation with flexibility. While having a birth plan is a great way to advocate for your preferences, it's equally important to stay open to the unexpected. Every childbirth experience is unique, even for mothers who have had multiple births, and being adaptable can help you navigate whatever comes your way.

Labor calls for both effort and release – strength and surrender.

Chapter 7
Health Tips While Pregnant

Your pregnancy journey is a time of incredible transformation, not just for your baby but for your own body as well. During this time, creating healthy foundations is one of the most empowering ways you can prepare for a vibrant pregnancy, a smoother labor, and a confident postpartum recovery. This chapter covers key areas of focus to help you nourish, strengthen, and support your body while also listening to its unique needs. From staying hydrated and managing discomforts to building your support team, these tips are designed to guide you through this remarkable stage of life.

Hydration

Pregnant women of all ages are recommended to drink at least 80 ounces, or 10 cups, of water each day. But hydration goes beyond just drinking water—it's about ensuring your body absorbs and uses it effectively. Adding electrolytes like sodium and potassium helps your cells retain this hydration. Some women find that adding a single crystal of Celtic salt to their water or incorporating electrolyte powders into their routine does the trick.

I regularly recommend premium electrolytes to my patients and emphasize the importance of choosing high-quality products. Brands that use well-sourced sea salt, such as Redmond's Real Salt, avoid heavy metal contaminants and provide a natural mineral boost. Another favorite is the adrenal cocktail, a simple mix of sodium, potassium, and whole food vitamin C, which supports your adrenals, energy levels, and hydration all at once. Keep in mind that stress, especially during pregnancy, can deplete magnesium—a vital mineral we'll discuss in the nutrition section.

Constipation

Constipation is a common challenge during pregnancy, but small, consistent habits can make a big difference. Staying hydrated, incorporating daily movement, and eating fiber-rich foods can keep things moving. Aim to sit on the toilet at a consistent time each day, ideally within 30 minutes of your first meal.

One natural and effective solution is kiwi fruit—eating two kiwis a day has been shown to outperform common remedies like psyllium husk and Miralax. Packed with soluble and insoluble fiber, kiwis are gentle on the digestive system and a great addition to your diet. Taking 5 slow belly breaths while sitting on the toilet can also help regulate bowel movements and calm your nervous system.

In postpartum, preventing constipation becomes even more essential to protect a healing pelvic floor. While stool softeners are often recommended in hospitals, alternatives like prunes or kiwis can be equally effective. If you need more support, consider magnesium citrate or probiotics, but always consult with your healthcare provider for personalized advice. Coping with constipation can be frustrating, but self-compassion and proactive care go a long way.

Daily Movement

Continuing regular movement during pregnancy is vital for maintaining physical and mental well-being. Whether it's walking, yoga, or another form of exercise that feels good for your body, daily activity has profound benefits:

- **Promotes Overall Health:** Improves cardiovascular fitness, strengthens muscles, and reduces risks like gestational diabetes or preeclampsia.

- **Boosts Mood:** Exercise releases endorphins, reducing stress and improving mood.

- **Prepares for Labor:** Strengthens the core and pelvic floor muscles needed for childbirth.

- **Supports Recovery:** Helps maintain fitness for an easier postpartum recovery.

Remember to listen to your body. For some women, running or high-intensity workouts feel great throughout pregnancy; for others, modifications may be necessary as symptoms like hip or pelvic pain arise. It's okay to adapt as your body changes.

Good Shoes and Arch Support

As the hormone relaxin increases during pregnancy, the ligaments in your body—including those in your feet—become looser. This can lead to discomfort or even changes in shoe size. Invest in high-quality footwear with arch support to prevent pain and long-term changes to the structure of your feet. Look for sandals or shoes designed for plantar fasciitis, especially if you're expecting in warmer months. And if your feet do stretch postpartum, don't worry—you can strengthen those muscles and return to your pre-pregnancy size!

Listening to Your Body

Pregnancy is a time to truly connect with your body. Whether it's reminding yourself to rest when you've been on your feet too long, hydrating when your baby's movements feel slower, or adjusting your fitness routine to prevent pain, learning to listen to your body's signals is a key skill. Your body knows what it needs—your job is to tune in and respond with care.

Find Your Support Team

Having a supportive and communicative team is essential for feeling empowered throughout pregnancy, birth, and postpartum. Make sure you feel comfortable with your healthcare providers and that they respect your preferences and informed choices. In addition to your OB-GYN or midwife, consider including professionals like doulas, pelvic PTs, lactation consultants, and mental health therapists in your support network.

If you're unsure where to start, local moms' groups on social media can be a treasure trove of recommendations. Use the birth support team page at the front of this book to write down the providers you want to contact or include in your care.

Conclusion

Building a strong foundation during pregnancy doesn't have to be overwhelming. By focusing on hydration, nutrition, movement, and support, you're giving your body and mind the tools they need for a healthy pregnancy and postpartum journey. Remember, these tips are meant to guide and empower you—not to add pressure. Take it one step at a time, and trust that the small, consistent habits you build now will have lasting benefits for you and your baby.

Nourishment isn't just food—it's movement, hydration, and listening to my body.

Chapter 8
Nutrition Essentials During Pregnancy and Postpartum

Nutrition is the foundation of a healthy pregnancy and postpartum recovery. While many women focus on meeting basic nutrient needs, key elements like protein, magnesium, healthy fats, and hydration are often overlooked. These nutrients play a vital role in supporting both your well-being and your baby's development. This section will cover the essentials, guiding you to feel strong, energized, and well-prepared for the transformative journey through pregnancy, postpartum, and beyond.

Protein: Your Body's Building Block

Protein is essential for both you and your baby. It plays a role in building the baby's tissues and organs, supporting muscle health, and stabilizing your blood sugar levels. During pregnancy, adequate protein intake can help balance energy and reduce the risk of gestational diabetes, especially when paired with healthy fats.

- **Protein and Bone Health:** Protein is crucial for bone strength and structure, providing the framework for strong bones. It aids in calcium absorption, promotes insulin-like growth factor (IGF-1) production (a key factor for bone health), and supports muscle mass, which in turn protects bone density.

- **Postpartum & Beyond:** Protein continues to play a key role postpartum, supporting tissue repair, muscle recovery, and hormonal balance. Research also shows that a protein-rich breakfast can dramatically reduce hunger throughout the day, helping to manage appetite and energy levels. In one study, teens who ate oatmeal for breakfast consumed 80% more calories throughout the day compared to those who had an omelet, despite both meals having the same number of calories.

Magnesium: The Miracle Mineral

Magnesium is critical for many processes in the body, including cellular function, energy production, and hormone balance. According to magnesium researcher Mildred Seelig, "Pregnancy is a magnesium-deficient state." Magnesium supports the function of enzymes in the uterus and helps prevent common pregnancy complications. Getting enough magnesium during pregnancy can help reduce the risk of:

- Leg cramps

- Preterm labor

- Morning sickness

- Low birth weight

- High blood pressure

- Fatigue

- Gestational diabetes

- Postpartum depression

How Much Magnesium Do You Need?

For most women, aiming for around **500 mg per day** of magnesium is ideal. During pregnancy, the body's demand increases, with estimates of at least **5-6 mg per pound of body weight**. Magnesium can be found in foods like spinach, almonds, and avocados, but it's often difficult to meet daily needs through food alone. Many women choose to supplement with magnesium glycinate or magnesium malate, which are more bioavailable forms of magnesium. Many studies have used the dose of 365 mg/day as the oral supplementation amount with positive results in maternal health and symptoms for all studies. If they are eating a well balanced diet, they are likely getting at least another 150mg from food for a total of at least 500mg/day.

Note: magnesium is a nutrient, not a medication. If a person is taking more than their body needs on any given day, their bowel movements will become more loose. This is a good indicator that a person can reduce their supplemental magnesium intake.

- **Magnesium Citrate:** While magnesium citrate is commonly used, it is primarily effective for relieving constipation by drawing water into the stool. It should not be taken as a primary source of magnesium for general health, as it is not as beneficial for muscle relaxation, energy production, or hormone regulation as magnesium glycinate or malate.

- **Gut Sensitivity and Magnesium:** Some women may experience gut sensitivity when taking oral magnesium supplements, particularly if they have a leaky gut or sensitive digestive system. In this case, magnesium can be applied topically through magnesium lotion or oil, which allows the body to absorb the nutrient through the skin. Over time, you can work with your holistic or functional medicine provider to gradually increase your oral intake.

Healthy Fats and Omega-3s: Essential for You and Baby

Healthy fats are vital during pregnancy and postpartum, especially omega-3 fatty acids like DHA and EPA, which support your baby's brain and eye development. Omega-3s also reduce inflammation and can help balance your mood postpartum, reducing the risk of postpartum depression.

Sources of Healthy Fats:

- **Fatty fish** like salmon and sardines (for omega-3s)
- **Chia seeds and flaxseeds** (for plant-based omega-3s)
- **Avocados, olive oil, and nuts** provide monounsaturated fats that support heart health and hormone production.

Healthy fats also aid in the absorption of fat-soluble vitamins like A, D, E, and K, making them an essential part of a balanced diet.

Folate and Choline: Vital for Baby's Development

Folate is essential for preventing neural tube defects in your baby, while choline supports brain development and overall cellular function. Many women are aware of the importance of folate, but choline is often overlooked, despite its critical role during pregnancy.

Sources of Folate:

- Leafy greens like spinach and kale

- Lentils and beans

Sources of Choline:

- **Eggs** (especially the yolks)

- **Beef liver** (also a great source of iron)

- **Chicken**

Both folate and choline can be obtained from a balanced diet, but many prenatal vitamins include folate in the form of folic acid, which can be harder for some women to metabolize. Opt for folate over folic acid whenever possible, and ensure you're getting over **500 mg of choline** daily, as many prenatal vitamins do not include enough choline.

Vitamin D and Calcium: For Strong Bones and Beyond

Vitamin D and calcium are two nutrients that work together to support bone health for both you and your baby. Calcium is essential for building strong bones and teeth, while vitamin D helps the body absorb calcium more efficiently.

Natural Sources of Vitamin D:

- **Sunlight**: Try to spend time outdoors for natural vitamin D production.

- **Fatty fish** like salmon and mackerel

- **Egg yolks** and dairy products

Calcium-Rich Foods:

- **Dairy products** like yogurt, milk, and cheese

- **Leafy greens** like kale and collard greens

- **Almonds and chia seeds** While calcium is often associated with bone health, it also plays a role in regulating muscle contractions and nerve function.

Hydration and Electrolyte Balance: Staying Hydrated for You and Baby

Drinking enough water is crucial during pregnancy and postpartum, but maintaining proper electrolyte balance is equally important. Electrolytes like sodium, potassium, calcium, and magnesium help regulate fluid levels, support muscle function, and reduce swelling.

Adrenal Cocktail: One simple way to stay hydrated while supporting electrolyte balance is through an adrenal cocktail. This can help nourish your adrenal glands, which are under extra stress during pregnancy. A typical adrenal cocktail contains:

- 4 oz. orange juice (for vitamin C and potassium)

- 1/4 tsp. cream of tartar (for potassium)

- 1/4 tsp. sea salt (for sodium)

This refreshing drink helps maintain hydration while also supporting your body's stress response. I often use a powdered adrenal cocktail mix that contains mineral salts, potassium, and whole-food vitamin C. I'll add it to a small amount of orange juice, or if I want to avoid the extra sugar, I mix it into water with a few drops of stevia. Another option is to look for powdered adrenal cocktail blends from reputable supplement companies that are made without fillers or added sweeteners. For links to my favorite trusted resources, see the **Birth Ready Bundle**.

Fiber: Supporting Digestive Health

Constipation is a common issue during pregnancy due to hormonal changes and the pressure on your digestive system. A diet rich in fiber can help keep things moving, reduce bloating, and improve overall gut health.

High-Fiber Foods to Include:

- **Fruits** like apples, berries, and pears

- **Vegetables** like broccoli and carrots

- **Whole grains** like oats, quinoa, and brown rice

- **Legumes** like lentils and chickpeas

Pairing fiber-rich foods with plenty of water will support smooth digestion and help prevent discomfort.

Supplementation: What to Look For in Prenatal Vitamins

Choosing the right prenatal vitamin is essential for supporting both your health and your baby's development. While supplements can help fill nutritional gaps, it's always ideal to prioritize whole food-based sources of nutrients whenever possible. Whole food nutrients are often more easily absorbed and utilized by the body, making them a superior option for many expecting mothers.

If swallowing pills is a challenge, consider prenatal vitamins available in powder form or smaller capsules. These options can make supplementation easier while ensuring you still get the nutrients you need.

Key Considerations for Prenatal Supplementation

- **Magnesium**: Look for at least 300 mg of magnesium in your prenatal vitamin. If the amount is lower, consider supplementing with magnesium glycinate or malate separately. These forms are highly bioavailable and support overall health better than magnesium citrate, which is more commonly used for constipation.

- **Choline**: Many prenatal vitamins lack adequate amounts of choline, a critical nutrient for fetal brain development and maternal liver health. Aim for over 500 mg daily, either through food sources or additional supplementation.

- **Folate (Not Folic Acid)**: Ensure your prenatal contains folate rather than folic acid. Folate is the natural form of this vitamin and is essential for preventing neural tube defects and supporting healthy development. Many people struggle to metabolize folic acid, making folate the superior choice.

- **Omega-3s or Cod Liver Oil**: For DHA and EPA, take a high-quality omega-3 supplement or cod liver oil separately from your prenatal vitamin. These nutrients are vital for brain and eye development, but they cannot be effectively included in most multivitamin formulas.

- **Whole Food-Based Options (Beef Liver Capsules)**: Organic beef liver capsules are an excellent example of whole food-based supplementation. Often called "nature's multivitamin," beef liver is packed with over 50 essential minerals, including bioavailable copper and retinol (vitamin A). Adding beef liver capsules to your regimen ensures your body receives these nutrients in their most natural and effective form.

The Right Prenatal for You

A high-quality prenatal vitamin, combined with targeted supplements like omega-3s, beef liver capsules, and magnesium, will help ensure you're meeting your body's unique needs during pregnancy and postpartum. Exploring powder or capsule options can also make it easier to stay consistent if traditional pills are difficult to take.

Teas for Pregnancy

If you enjoy tea, certain herbal blends can offer nutritional and calming benefits. These teas not only hydrate but also address common pregnancy concerns:

- **Peppermint Tea**: Eases digestion and reduces nausea.

- **Ginger Tea**: Combats nausea and digestive discomfort.

- **Nettle Tea**: Rich in iron, calcium, and magnesium, supporting muscle health and vitality.

- **Chamomile Tea**: Promotes relaxation and reduces stress.

- **Raspberry Leaf Tea**: May strengthen uterine muscles for labor preparation. Consult your provider before use.

- **Lemon Balm Tea**: Helps ease anxiety and promote calmness.

Conclusion

Good nutrition is a powerful way to support both your health and your baby's development during pregnancy and postpartum. By focusing on essential nutrients—protein, magnesium, healthy fats, folate, and choline—and staying hydrated, you're setting the foundation for a vibrant journey. For added benefits, incorporate herbal teas that soothe, nourish, and complement your overall wellness routine.

Chapter 9
Prenatal Exercises

There are countless mobility and strength exercises out there—but you don't need a complicated routine to feel strong and supported during pregnancy. In this section, I've chosen a few that cover the essentials and can be done with little to no equipment, making them realistic to fit into daily life.

For **mobility,** I encourage you to try each exercise and notice how your body responds. Choose the ones that feel most helpful and keep coming back to those—you don't need to do the entire flow every time. The goal is to release tension, create space, and prepare your body with ease.

For **strength,** you'll find a couple of simple movements that target your core, upper body, hips, and legs. If you're already following a strength program you enjoy, keep at it. But on busy days when carving out 20–60 minutes isn't possible, this flow still counts. Small, consistent movement makes a difference.

These exercises aren't about perfection or intensity. They're about building strength where you need it most, creating mobility where it matters, and giving yourself permission to do what's realistic. With breath as your foundation, these simple movements will support you through pregnancy, labor, and into postpartum recovery.

Prenatal Exercises

Mobility Exercises

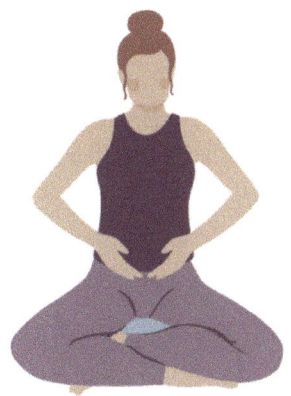

Belly Breathing:
Place your hands on your belly and chest. Slowly inhale through your nose and allow your belly to expand (not shoulders or chest), exhale through softly pursed lips and let belly recoil. Can also place hands on ribs to cue inhaling into ribs.

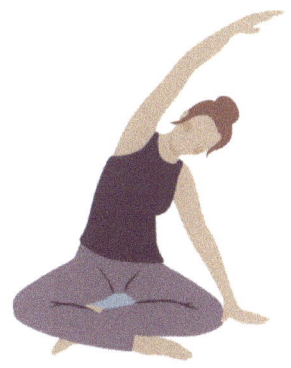

Seated Side Bend:
Sitting on yoga block with legs crossed, place one hand to the side and reach the other arm overhead to the side. Take 2-3 slow inhales focused on expanding the lengthened side of your body before switching to the other side.

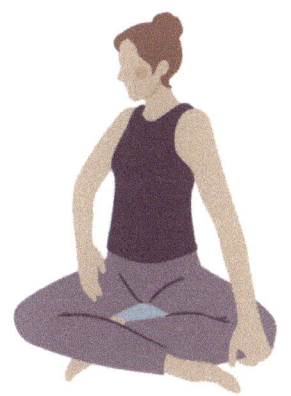

Seated Spine Twist:
Sitting on yoga block with legs crossed, rotate spine using hands to support this twist. Take 2-3 slow inhales focused on letting your ribcage to expand softly.

Prenatal Exercises

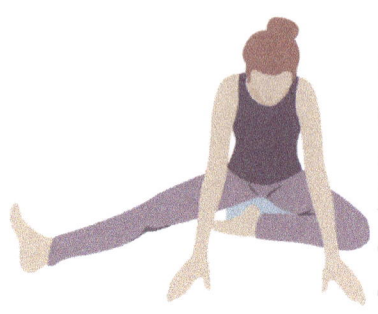

Inner Thigh Stretch:
Sit on a yoga block or a firm cushion. Bend one leg and stretch the other leg out to the side. Keep your back straight and slowly lean forward until you feel a gentle stretch on the inside of your thigh. Take 2–3 slow, deep breaths and relax into the stretch.

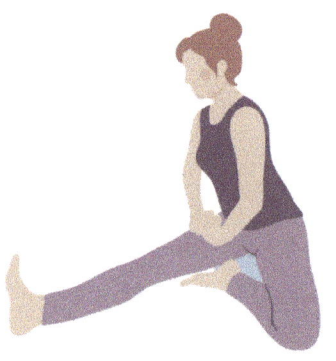

Hamstring Stretch:
Sit tall on one or two yoga blocks. Stretch one leg straight out in front of you and keep your back straight. Gently lean forward toward your foot until you feel a light stretch in the back of your leg. Take 2–3 slow, deep breaths and relax into the stretch.

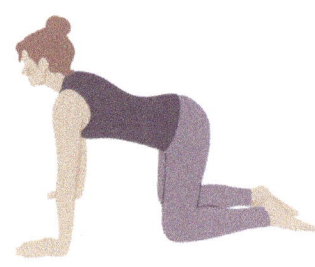
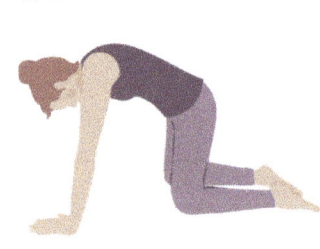

Cat-Cow Stretch:
Start on your hands and knees with your wrists under your shoulders and knees under your hips.

As you inhale, let your belly drop down, untuck your tailbone, and lift your head.

As you exhale, round your back, tuck your tailbone, and bring your chin toward your chest.

Move slowly between these two positions, matching your breath. Repeat for about 5 rounds of slow, steady breathing.

Prenatal Exercises

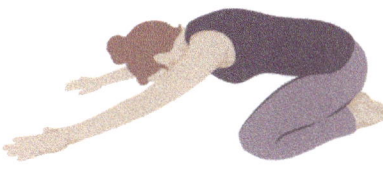

Child's Pose:
Start on your hands and knees. Gently sit your hips back toward your feet as you stretch your arms forward. Take slow breaths into your lower back and pelvis. You can place a pillow behind your knees if it feels more comfortable. Stay in this position for 4–5 slow, deep breaths.

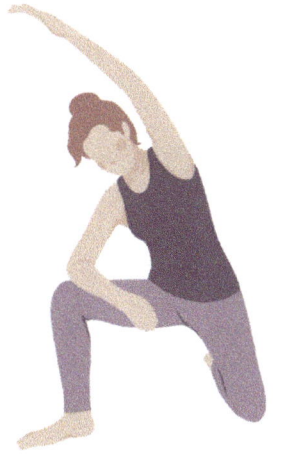

Kneeling Pelvic Opener:
Start with one knee on the floor and the other foot stepped out to the side on a diagonal. Gently shift your weight toward the front foot until you feel a stretch in your inner thighs. You can reach one arm overhead to add a side stretch. Take 3 slow, deep breaths, then switch sides and repeat.

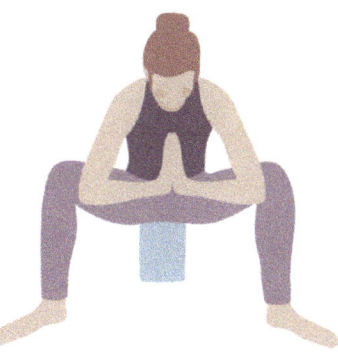

Supported Squat:
Sit on a low stool or sturdy surface with your feet wide apart and your back tall. Lean forward slightly and rest your elbows between your knees, pressing your hands together for support. As you breathe in, let your belly relax and drop. Continue for 5–10 slow, steady breaths.

Prenatal Exercises

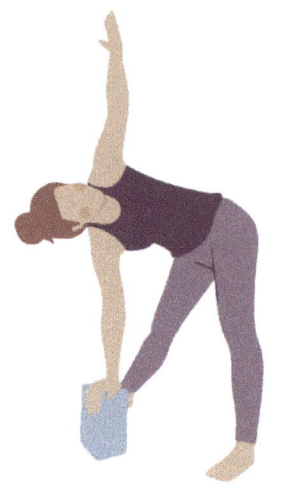

Modified Windmill:
Stand with your feet wide and toes pointing forward. Hinge forward at your hips and place your hands on a block, chair, or desk for support. Gently twist your upper body and reach one arm up toward the ceiling while bending the knee on that same side into a small lunge. Take 2–3 slow breaths, then return to center and switch sides.
(This stretch helps open the inner thighs, hamstrings, and spine, and also supports gentle sciatic nerve mobility.)

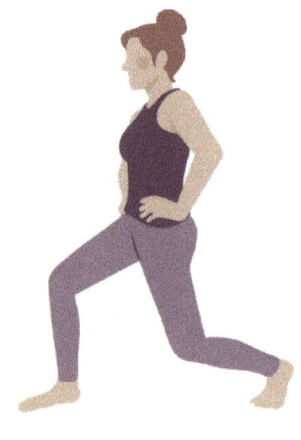

Hip Flexor Stretch:
Stand with one foot in front of the other. Keep your back straight and gently tuck your tailbone under. Shift your weight toward your front foot until you feel a stretch in the front of your back hip. Take 3 slow, deep breaths.
(You can also place your front foot on a low step or sturdy chair for a deeper stretch.)

Prenatal Exercises

Strength Exercises

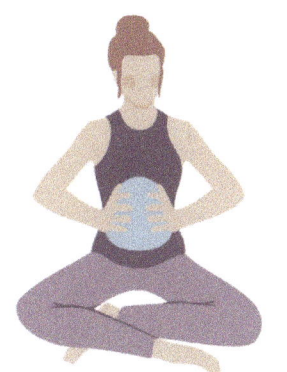

Seated Core Brace:

Sit tall on a yoga block or chair and hold a small Pilates ball or soft ball between your hands with your elbows wide. Take a deep breath in to prepare. As you exhale, press into the ball and gently draw your belly in toward your spine. Repeat for 5 slow breaths, then relax and repeat as needed.

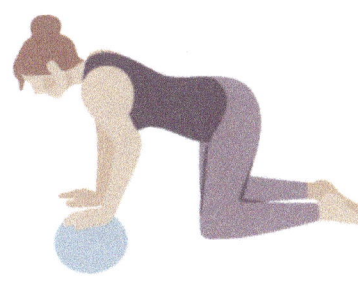

Hands and Knees Core Brace:

Start on your hands and knees with a Pilates ball or soft ball under one hand. As you inhale, let your belly relax and drop slightly. As you exhale, press your hand downward onto the ball and draw your belly toward your spine to engage your core. Repeat for 5 slow breaths on each side.

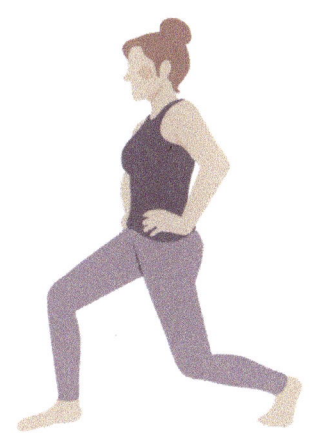

Staggered Stance Lunge:

Stand tall with one foot in front of the other. Keep your spine straight as you slowly bend your back knee to lower your body down. You can do a shallow lunge or bring your back knee close to the floor. Move with your breath—inhale as you lower and exhale as you return to standing. Start with 6–8 repetitions and work up to 10–15 as you get stronger.

Prenatal Exercises

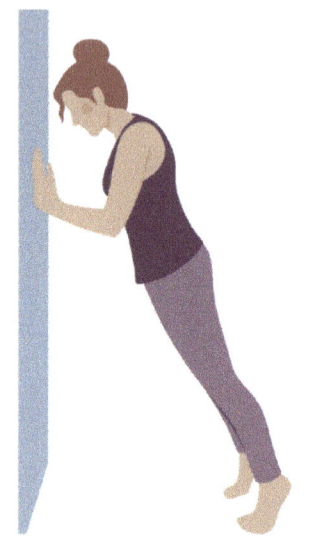

Incline Push Ups:
(use wall or kitchen counter)

Stand facing a wall or kitchen counter and place your hands slightly wider than your shoulders. Keep your weight on the balls of your feet, squeeze your glutes, and draw your shoulder blades and front ribs down to set your core. Inhale as you lower your chest toward the counter, then exhale as you press back up. Start with 6–8 repetitions and work up to 10–15 as you get stronger.

Booty Taps / Mini Squats:

Stand about 12 inches in front of a wall or the arm of a couch with your feet hip-width apart and your palms together. You can place a resistance loop band around your knees for an extra glute challenge.

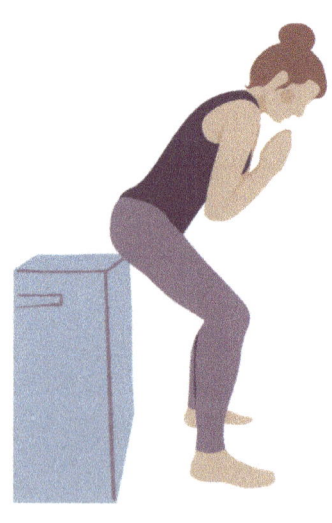

Hinge your hips back first, then gently bend your knees while pressing your knees slightly outward. Keep your spine tall and your core engaged. Inhale as you lower until your bottom lightly taps the wall or a chair, and exhale as you return to standing. You should feel this mostly in your glutes—not your back or hip flexors. Perform 10–20 repetitions.

Tips on Fitting in Exercises: Habit Stacking

Find ways to slip in exercises by stacking them with other daily habits. I call this Habit Stacking. Instead of thinking that we always need to carve out large chunks of time for exercises and self-care, break things up so that they actually get done and you can feel like you are winning at the self-care game.

Habit Stacking Examples:

- Take 5 belly breaths every toilet trip.

- Do a few kitchen counter push-ups and lunges while waiting for coffee to brew or water to boil.

- Take a chair stretch break when sitting at your desk while working or scrolling social media.

- Do a favorite stretch before getting into bed.

- Practice pelvic floor "let go" breathing while brushing your teeth.

- Stand on one foot at a time while washing dishes to improve balance and hip strength.

- Use the time spent folding laundry to do gentle squats or pelvic tilts.

- Squeeze in calf raises while brushing your hair or putting on makeup.

- Take a minute to stretch your arms overhead and twist side to side when unloading the dishwasher.

- Walk around the house or perform gentle stretches during phone calls.

Tips for Success

- **Start Small**: Pick one or two habits to stack initially, and build from there. Consistency is more important than quantity.

- **Set Visual Reminders**: Place a sticky note or an object, like a yoga mat or resistance band, near areas where you'll perform the habit stack.

- **Use Timers**: Set gentle reminders on your phone or a smart device to integrate habit stacks into your day.

- **Celebrate Wins**: Acknowledge your efforts, no matter how small they feel. Every habit stack is a step toward your self-care goals.

Homework: Your Action Steps Each Week

Creating small, consistent habits now will set the foundation for a smoother birth and recovery. These steps are designed to be simple, approachable, and easy to integrate into your daily life. Remember, the goal isn't perfection—it's progress!

Here's what to focus on:

1. **Daily Belly Breathing**: Spend 5–10 minutes practicing belly breathing. *Habit Stack*: Do this while lying in bed before you fall

asleep or after you wake up in the morning.

2. **Pelvic Floor Connection**: On your INHALE, focus on gently lengthening your pelvic floor as you breathe in. *Tip*: Lie on your side and place the fingers of your top hand just inside your top sit bone (ischial tuberosity). As you inhale, feel for the gentle expansion or bulging of your pelvic floor muscles. Don't worry about perfection—this is about building awareness and connection.

3. **Core Prenatal Exercises**: Commit to doing your prenatal exercises at least 3 times before reading the next section. *Habit Stack*: Pair this with another activity like watching your favorite show or waiting for dinner to cook.

Consistency Over Perfection

Take it one day at a time—these small steps add up to big progress. If you miss a day, no problem! Pick up where you left off and keep going. The most important thing is to create a rhythm that works for you.

Preparation isn't about doing everything perfectly—it's about starting small and staying consistent.

Chapter 10
Self-Care Challenge By Trimester
Self-Care Assessments, Goals, & Self-Care Bingos

PREGNANCY IS A TIME of incredible transformation—not just for your body, but for your mind, emotions, and relationships. While much of the focus tends to be on preparing for your baby, it's equally important to care for **you**. By nurturing yourself, you're not only supporting your own well-being but also creating a stronger, more balanced foundation for motherhood.

This section is designed to help you keep your well-being front and center throughout your pregnancy. Each trimester comes with its own unique challenges and opportunities, which is why this self-care challenge is tailored to meet you where you are, no matter how far along you may be.

What to Expect in Each Trimester's Challenge

1. **Self-Care Assessment:** Begin each trimester by reflecting on your self-care habits. Use the simple 1–5 scale to evaluate how you're caring for your **mind, body,** and **relationships**. This isn't about being perfect—it's about gaining clarity on where you're thriving and where you might want to give yourself a little more love.

2. **Self-Care Goals:** Next, set meaningful self-care goals for the trimester. Choose from suggested ideas or add your own, and think about how small, consistent actions can make a big difference in your overall well-being.

3. **Self-Care Challenge Bingo:** Finally, dive into the interactive Bingo-style self-care challenge! Each card includes 30 simple, nourishing activities, from taking a magnesium bath to watching a sunset. As you check off each square, you'll create intentional moments of joy, relaxation, and connection. Whether you complete a row, a column, or the whole card, the goal is to have fun while putting your well-being first.

Why Self-Care Matters During Pregnancy

Taking care of yourself during pregnancy isn't a luxury—it's essential. By prioritizing your mind, body, and relationships, you're not only preparing for the demands of birth and parenthood but also embracing the unique journey of pregnancy. This challenge invites you to pause, reflect, and take action to support the whole person you are.

So grab your pen, dive in, and remember: the better you care for yourself, the better equipped you'll be to care for the little one growing inside you. Let's make self-care a habit that lasts well beyond pregnancy.

First Trimester
Self-Care Assessment

Rate each area to help you focus on your well being this trimester. 1 means you are not satisfied with where you are and need things to change and 5 means you are happy with where you are.

MIND:
My overall well-being. I allow time to recharge, am safe from burn out, feel present and focused.

① ② ③ ④ ⑤

BODY:
I choose healthy foods, make time for walks/exercise, drink enough water, sleep, listen to my body.

① ② ③ ④ ⑤

MY RELATIONSHIPS:
I feel supported, show love to others,, spend quality time with my loved one/s, communicate my needs.

① ② ③ ④ ⑤

Notes:

First Trimester Self-Care Goals

Each season of pregnancy invites new ways to care for your whole self. Take a moment to reflect on what matters most right now. Use this page to set 1–3 goals in each area—Mind, Body, and Relationships—to help you feel grounded, supported, and well. (Need inspiration? See examples beside each section.)

GOALS FOR MY MIND:

<u>Mental Health</u>
- Mindfulness
- Journaling
- Decluttering

<u>Spiritual</u>
- Gratitude
- Meditation/Prayer

GOALS FOR MY BODY:

- Rest
- Daily walks
- Healthy Foods
- Meet protein goals
- Water
- Prenatal Exercises
- Sleep
- Breathing Practice

GOALS FOR MY RELATIONSHIPS:

- Communication
- Quality time
- Feeling Connected
- Date nights
- Meeting each other's needs

First Trimester Self-Care Bingo

Self-care doesn't have to be big or fancy—small moments count. Use this bingo card as a gentle reminder to care for yourself in simple ways. Check off what you've already done or circle what you'd like to try next. There's no right way to play—just notice what helps you feel good and supported.

Stretch your body	Drink more water	Go for a walk	Eat a treat	Go to bed early
Write a bucket list	Listen to your favorite music	Take a magnesium bath	Buy yourself a gift	Spend time with a friend
Practice yoga	Journal	Have an electrolyte drink	Make a gratitude list	Write a letter to your younger self
Watch a sunrise	Read or listen to a book	Watch a favorite movie	Visit a new coffee shop or restaurant	Get your nails done
Spend time in the sun	Take your magnesium	Say "no" to something that drains you	Relax with legs up the wall	Make yourself a protein smoothie
Take a nap	Babymoon	Find a guided meditation you like	Watch the sunset	Read affirmations

Second Trimester Self-Care Assessment

Rate each area to help you focus on your well being this trimester. 1 means you are not satisfied with where you are and need things to change and 5 means you are happy with where you are.

MIND:
My overall well-being. I allow time to recharge, am safe from burn out, feel present and focused.

1 2 3 4 5

BODY:
I choose healthy foods, make time for walks/exercise, drink enough water, sleep, listen to my body.

1 2 3 4 5

MY RELATIONSHIPS:
I feel supported, show love to others,, spend quality time with my loved one/s, communicate my needs.

1 2 3 4 5

Notes:

Second Trimester Self-Care Goals

Each season of pregnancy invites new ways to care for your whole self. Take a moment to reflect on what matters most right now. Use this page to set 1–3 goals in each area—Mind, Body, and Relationships—to help you feel grounded, supported, and well. (Need inspiration? See examples beside each section.)

GOALS FOR MY MIND:

<u>Mental Health</u>
- Mindfulness
- Journaling
- Decluttering

<u>Spiritual</u>
- Gratitude
- Meditation/Prayer

GOALS FOR MY BODY:

- Rest
- Daily walks
- Healthy Foods
- Meet protein goals
- Water
- Prenatal Exercises
- Sleep
- Breathing Practice

GOALS FOR MY RELATIONSHIPS:

- Communication
- Quality time
- Feeling Connected
- Date nights
- Meeting each other's needs

Second Trimester Self-Care Bingo

Self-care doesn't have to be big or fancy—small moments count. Use this bingo card as a gentle reminder to care for yourself in simple ways. Check off what you've already done or circle what you'd like to try next. There's no right way to play—just notice what helps you feel good and supported.

Move your body	Drink more water	Go for a walk with your partner or friend	Call a friend who makes you laugh	Go to bed early
Prep healthy snacks ahead of time	Listen to your favorite music	Take a magnesium bath	Buy yourself a gift	Spend time with a friend
Practice yoga	Have an electrolyte drink	Write 3 things you're grateful for	Drink a glass of water before checking your phone	Take a nap without guilt
Watch a sunrise/sunset	Read a book	Watch a favorite movie	Visit a new coffee shop or restaurant	Get your nails done
Spend time in the sun	Take your magnesium	Organize your closet	Relax with legs up the wall	Make yourself a protein smoothie
Take a nap	Babymoon	Find a guided meditation you like	Watch the sunset	Write an affirmation that you need right now

Third Trimester
Self-Care Assessment

Rate each area to help you focus on your well being this trimester. 1 means you are not satisfied with where you are and need things to change and 5 means you are happy with where you are.

MIND:
My overall well-being. I allow time to recharge, am safe from burn out, feel present and focused.

BODY:
I choose healthy foods, make time for walks/exercise, drink enough water, sleep, listen to my body.

MY RELATIONSHIPS:
I feel supported, show love to others,, spend quality time with my loved one/s, communicate my needs.

Notes:

Third Trimester Self-Care Goals

Each season of pregnancy invites new ways to care for your whole self. Take a moment to reflect on what matters most right now. Use this page to set 1–3 goals in each area—Mind, Body, and Relationships—to help you feel grounded, supported, and well. (Need inspiration? See examples beside each section.)

GOALS FOR MY MIND:

<u>Mental Health</u>
- Mindfulness
- Journaling
- Decluttering

<u>Spiritual</u>
- Gratitude
- Meditation/Prayer

GOALS FOR MY BODY:

- Rest
- Daily walks
- Healthy Foods
- Meet protein goals
- Water
- Prenatal Exercises
- Sleep
- Breathing Practice

GOALS FOR MY RELATIONSHIPS:

- Communication
- Quality time
- Feeling Connected
- Date nights
- Meeting each other's needs

Third Trimester Self-Care Bingo

Self-care doesn't have to be big or fancy—small moments count. Use this bingo card as a gentle reminder to care for yourself in simple ways. Check off what you've already done or circle what you'd like to try next. There's no right way to play—just notice what helps you feel good and supported.

Stretch your body	Drink more water	Go for a walk	Buy yourself fresh flowers	Go to bed early
Get a massage	Listen to your favorite music	Take a magnesium bath	Get a pedicure	Spend time with a friend
Practice yoga or other relaxing movement	Say "no" to something that drains you	Have an electrolyte drink	Soak your feet in epsom salt	Listen to a favorite song with eyes closed
Watch a sunrise	Read a book	Watch a favorite show	Visit a new coffee shop or restaurant	Buy something just for you
Spend time in the sun	Take your magnesium	Diffuse your favorite essential oil	Elevate your legs and have a hydrating drink	Get breakfast with a friend
Take a nap	Take 10 deep slow breaths before bed	Find a guided meditation you like	Watch the sunset	Read your affirmations

Every act of self-care is an act of preparation. I am worth the effort.

Every small step I take strengthens the foundation for my health and my baby's well-being.

Take this moment to pause, reflect, and honor the progress you've already made.

How do you feel about the journey you're on right now? What intentions can you set to nurture yourself as you continue forward?

Every small step I take strengthens the foundation for my health and my baby's well-being.

Reflect on what you've learned so far and how it's shaping your mindset.

What has surprised or inspired you about your body or health during this stage of pregnancy? How does this insight influence how you care for yourself moving forward?

Every small step I take strengthens the foundation for my health and my baby's well-being.

Reflect on what you've learned so far and how it's shaping your mindset.

What is one small, achievable step you can take this week to nurture your mind, body, or relationships?

Which area of your self-care—mind, body, or relationships—feels most in need of extra attention, and why?

SECTION II: Preparing to Push

For most expecting women, they have been told that childbirth is natural and that they will just "push" when they feel they should or when they are told to push. There will be many women that feel that pushing came to them intuitively and the pushing phase was easy for them. However, many women do not feel like they know what this means and very often will struggle to connect to their core and pelvic floor muscles to push effectively or even be at an increased risk of perineal tearing. How am I supposed to prepare to push?

This section covers *Preparing to Push:*

- Timeline For Birth Preparation

- The best labor positions

- Your glottis and your pelvic floor

- By week 30: Inversions and why we like all fours

- Preventing Perineal Tears

- Birth Coaching with Pelvic PTs or OTs

- Back and Belly Support: Taping vs braces for belly and back pain

- Homework Time

- Journal Pages For Birth Preparation

Chapter 11
How am I Supposed to Prepare to Push?

Why do women struggle to push?

As a PELVIC FLOOR therapist, I have found that the majority of patients over the years have had issues with having excessive tension in their pelvic floor muscles and truly struggled to relax or let go of the tension they have just at rest. This can lead to increased bladder irritation, bladder leaks and pain with sex or gynecological exams. Telling them initially to just "relax" their pelvic floor muscles is not helpful advice for them.

Even if this does not sound like you, know that many of my clients had no symptoms of feeling tension or pain… just occasional bladder leaks with activity or hard sneezes.

Women with this issue of tension have to slowly build the skills one at a time to first breathe well and relax tension in their belly to then be able to start working to reduce tension with their pelvic floor. For some, this can take a few weeks and others a few months depending on their circumstances.

This is why a self assessment at minimum or assessment by a skilled pelvic floor PT or OT is so helpful to pregnant women once they are in their second trimester or in the early 20's in weeks of gestation. Pushing requires us to *relax* and *let go* of tension in our pelvic floor muscles and coordinate our abdominal muscles to create a downward pressure with a contracting uterus to help our baby move through and out of the birth canal.

Preparing to push should include:

- A pelvic floor assessment to screen for any excess pelvic floor and hip tension that needs to be resolved before our due date.

- Learning and practicing effective breathing in coordination with our abdominal and pelvic floor muscles.

- Practicing multiple birth positions with pelvic breathing and working to release and bulge our pelvic floor muscles.

Preparation creates confidence. Confidence creates ease.

Chapter 12
Timeline for Birth Preparation

While there is no hard timeline for preparing for birth, the following is a loose guide for when we should ideally be working on certain elements of our birth preparation. You may be picking this book up before you are even pregnant or anytime during your pregnancy, so I wish for you to *not* feel stressed if you feel you have begun this journey too late. Realize that I have seen many women for birth coaching that were only a few weeks from their due date. Any birth prep is good birth prep! You are already so much more informed than most women at this point in time as the standard of care is zero birth prep besides packing a hospital bag and choosing a birth provider.

First Trimester

- Focusing on nourishing your body with healthy foods (organic if possible), staying hydrated (clean water and electrolytes) and choosing nutrients to support you with magnesium malate or glycinate being top of the list. (See nutrition section of this book!)

- Continuing healthy movement like walking most days or your exercise regimen as it works for your body.

- Prenatal prep exercises: focusing on connected breathing, hip, spinal, and pelvic mobility, maintaining core and hip strength

Second Trimester

- Pelvic Floor self assessment and find a pelvic floor PT or OT to be screened for any issues that may impede a smooth delivery and address any aches and pains during your pregnancy.

- Prenatal birth prep exercises multiple days/week

- Daily walks

- Daily breathing practice 5 minutes a day

- Working on relaxation techniques and finding things that make you feel calm and soothed such as essential oils you like, postures or stretches, calming music or binaural beats, guided meditations or affirmations that resonate with you.

- Continue focusing on nutrient dense foods, nutrients to support you and baby, and hydration with electrolytes daily.

Third Trimester

- By 30 weeks, getting into inversion postures and hands and knees daily to help with baby getting/staying head down.

- Prenatal prep exercises most days, both mobility and for pushing muscle strength (deep abdominals, upper body strength and squats; this could be as little as 5-10 minutes on busy days).

- Walking daily even for 5-10 minutes.

- Continue with nutrient dense foods and maintain good hydration, trace minerals (enzymes run the body and are made up of trace minerals), electrolyte (sodium and potassium) and magnesium (glycinate or malate for cells, mag citrate for temporary constipation support). This will help you with fatigue and muscle cramps!

- See your pelvic physical therapist for *any* issues with back or hip/pelvic pain and get support with back brace selection and even belly taping for support and pain relief.

- Push prep session/s with your pelvic therapist.

Find the positions that make me feel grounded yet supported and strong— they'll guide my birth journey.

Chapter 13
The Best Labor Positions

Babies are born to their mothers in multiple ways with mom in many different positions. It is important to know that there are great and not so great positions to birth which we will cover. But the *best* birth position for you is the one that feels *good* for you! We will get into how our position relates to the pelvis and what positions are best based on the stage of labor you are in. (Stage 1, transition, or stage 2)

As a pelvic PT, I must emphasize that the least favorable position, which many women end up in due to hospital routines and provider convenience, is lying on our backs with legs in stirrups. It's quite frustrating! Exploring the labor stages and ideal positions will highlight the inadequacy of this common posture for most women.

Pelvic Inlet

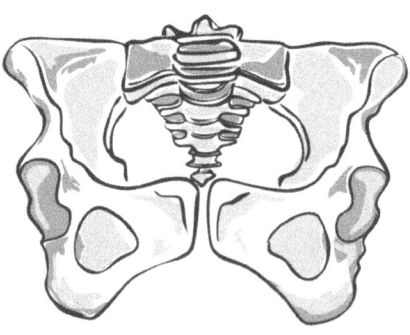

Pelvic Outlet

Stage One

This is the stage where you are in active labor and baby is beginning to engage in the pelvic inlet (the top of the pelvis). As our pelvic bones are primed to be a bit more relaxed (thanks to pregnancy hormones), they will actually be able to move to accommodate our baby.

Positions that will help the pelvic inlet widen can include:

- Hips outwardly rotated

- Knees wider than pelvis

- One or both knees higher than pelvis (flexed)

- Side lying with a peanut ball with top knee higher than ankle and hip outwardly rotated somewhat.

- Supported squat on ball, stool, or toilet.

- Standing side lunge with one leg on step or stool

- Reclined sitting with knees wider than hips

- Ensure that your lower back maintains a neutral or slightly rounded position, avoiding an excessive arch in the lumbar spine. This alignment helps create optimal space for the baby to engage with the pelvic inlet, as a flatter or gentle C-curve in the spine is more ideal.

Movements that can help baby move into the pelvis or descend further if stalled:

- Childs' pose with toes touching and knees wide. Slowly rock body forward over hands and back over heels. Focus on slow breaths and letting belly sag. (helps when baby is at top of pelvis to move into mid pelvis)

- Hands and knees rocking forward and back with one knee on a block, knees a bit wider than feet. (can help moving further down in pelvis)

- Feet side by side with one foot on stool or higher on a sturdy chair. Shifting weight out over the stool and back while breathing slowly while focusing on releasing tension. (helps baby move from mid pelvis to lower pelvis)

Stage Two

This is the Pushing Stage.

We hope that before we begin to actively push, that we actually *feel* the urge to push. This sometimes does not occur, especially in a medical setting. Pushing is *much* easier to do, when the body and mind has signaled that it is go time. When this happens, it can feel much more like we are merely assisting our body that is on autopilot.

Additionally, our birth provider can confirm with the birth providers that we are 10cm dilated and we are at zero stage or more, meaning that the baby has progressed down into our pelvis to where pushing can be effective.

At this stage, the baby has already moved through the pelvic inlet and is ready to transition out of the pelvic outlet. Positions that encourage our sit bones and tailbone at the outlet to open or separate from each other are most ideal. This would look quite the opposite from first stage positions. In the second stage, we want our hips to be more neutral for rotation and even slightly internally rotated. Being sure we are in a position that the tailbone is *not* tucked under us is also necessary.

Positions that will help widen the pelvic outlet can include:

- Hips neutral or internally rotated slightly

- Hands and knees (allows lots of freedom of movement for all pelvic bones and can relieve low back pressure). Using the CUB to support your body in hands and knees is a favorite of many of my patients.

- Side lying with top leg on bolster or peanut ball (not too much hip external/outward rotation)

- Kneeling in tub with knees only slightly apart

- Sitting upright on birthing stool (tailbone untucked/ leaning forearms on knees)

Note: If you end up needing to push while on your back or are more comfortable pushing in that position, you can use two rolled bath towels under each buttock lengthwise. This will help to free up the tailbone and sacrum to move down towards the bed, allowing the baby to navigate through the pelvic outlet more easily and protect your tailbone.

Chapter 14
The Glottis, Jaw, And The Pelvic Floor

IF YOU DIDN'T KNOW, our glottis (back of the throat) and jaw can impact whether our pelvic floor muscles are relaxed or grippy. Does this sound crazy to you? How about you try a couple of things...

What happens to your pelvic floor when you:

- Grip/tense your throat and hold your breath (Your pelvic floor likely tenses up)

- Relax your jaw and throat and blow through soft lips. (Your pelvic floor should relax)

- Say "Eeeee" high pitched (Your pelvic floor should tense up)

- Say "Huuuuuh" low pitched (Your pelvic floor should relax)

As you are not currently in labor, now is a good time to start noticing what you are doing with your neck and jaw. Do you find you tend to have tension in this area when focusing on something or stressed? If so, checking in with your body throughout the day to consciously work to relax your neck and jaw would be very helpful. And in labor, I recommend for birth partners to give a gentle reminder to their partner if they notice them tensing their jaw or neck.

Additionally, this is why we are *not* fans of holding our breath to push a baby out or when having a bowel movement for that matter. Both tasks require the pelvic floor to be relaxed and breath holding will make that all but impossible!

To Work On Now:

- Minimize forward head postures (increases jaw and neck strain)

- Use head rests (in car, watching TV, etc)

- Practice Resting Jaw Position 1) tongue resting at roof of mouth 2) teeth slightly apart 3) lips softly closed

- Break up longer stretches of reading, computer time with gentle rotations/wiggles of neck and jaw

During Labor:

- Good neck support

- Have a partner spot your jaw for tension

- Practicing breathing with a relaxed jaw

Chapter 15

By 30 Weeks; Inversions and Being on All Fours

Around the 30-week mark, providers typically begin checking to ensure the baby is positioned head down. This ideal positioning is crucial for birth, especially as the baby grows larger each week, making it harder for them to flip to the head-down position.

If the baby is not head down by 30 weeks, it is recommended that we get into quadruped (hands & knees) or inversion postures 3 times a day for 3-5 minutes each time.

Do them once a day if baby *is* head down, though note that hands and knees belly breathing is already in your prenatal exercises.

Option 1:

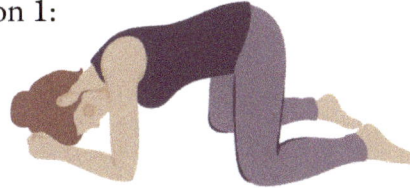

In either posture, focus on letting your belly drop towards the floor with each slow inhale to release any belly or pelvic tension.

Option 2:

Chapter 16
Preventing Perineal Tears

The thought of perineal tearing during birth can be a source of anxiety for many women—and that's completely normal. It's okay to feel concerned, but I want to reassure you: your body is designed to heal, and your birth team is there to care for you every step of the way. As a pelvic health specialist, I've worked with hundreds of women since 2010 who experienced perineal tears and went on to recover fully. While preventing a tear is an ideal goal, it's important to remember that if a tear does occur, healing is possible, and there are proactive steps you can take now to reduce your risk and support recovery.

Preparing the Perineum: Connection, Breath, and Release

Preparing your perineum for birth begins with connecting to your pelvic floor through breathwork. This connection is essential for effective pushing and protecting your perineum during labor. The goal is to learn to lengthen and release your pelvic floor muscles with each inhale and maintain that release during your exhale as you gently push. Coordinating this effort with your transverse abdominals and the natural contractions of your uterus can make a significant difference.

In my one-on-one birth coaching sessions, we often practice "zen" breathing, focusing solely on the breath until around week 34 or 35. As your due date approaches, we transition to practicing the coordination of releasing on the inhale and gently applying downward force on the exhale. Untucking your tailbone during the exhale can further release tension in the pelvic area—key for reducing strain during the pushing phase of labor.

Screening for Tension Before the Third Trimester

Ideally, it's best to begin screening for tension or tenderness in your pelvic floor before the third trimester. This gives you time to resolve any issues, ensuring your muscles are pliable and responsive by the time you give birth.

You can work with a pelvic floor PT or OT to identify and release areas of tension, but a self-assessment can also be helpful. Using a mirror and gently pressing on the muscles around your vaginal opening, ask yourself:

- Does the tissue feel soft and pliable, or tense and resistant?
- Are there any tender areas?
- Can you release tension by taking slow, deep breaths and focusing on gently bulging the muscles outward?

If you notice areas of tightness or tenderness, consult with a pelvic floor therapist for guidance. Remember—tense pelvic floor muscles don't guarantee a tear, just as relaxed muscles don't guarantee an intact perineum. Every birth is unique.

Is Perineal Massage Helpful?

Research shows that starting perineal massage around 35 weeks can reduce the risk of tearing during birth. However, this is just one part of the preparation process. Massage helps by increasing awareness, reducing muscle tension, and improving tissue pliability.

Self-massage can be performed with a finger, thumb, or a pelvic wand like the Intimate Rose wand. The key is to work with your breath: as you inhale, gently stretch the muscles and focus on relaxing your pelvic floor. Avoid applying excessive pressure, which can cause strain.

A pelvic floor PT or OT can guide you in performing perineal massage effectively. If you're finding it difficult to reach certain areas, they may recommend tools or provide hands-on guidance to help you prepare.

How We Push Matters

How you push during labor can significantly influence the risk of tearing. Open-glottis pushing—exhaling gently as you push—has been shown to reduce the risk of tearing, especially when combined with optimal labor positions.

Unfortunately, many women are still instructed to hold their breath and push in 10-second intervals. This outdated approach can cause unnecessary tension in the pelvic floor and reduce oxygen flow to both you and your baby.

When you understand how to connect your breath with your core and pelvic floor, you create the best conditions for effective pushing. Remember:

Powerful Pushing = Connecting to Your Core and Pelvic Floor + Effective Labor Positions + Breathing With Your Pushes.

Birth Providers' Role in Reducing Tears

Your birth provider plays a key role in helping protect your perineum during the second stage of labor. Applying warm compresses to the perineum can increase blood flow, soften tissues, and promote elasticity.

They may also provide valuable feedback during pushing, encouraging you to slow down if your perineum needs more time to stretch. This controlled pacing allows the tissues to adapt gradually, reducing the likelihood of trauma and contributing to a safer, more comfortable delivery.

What If Baby Comes Too Fast?

Sometimes, babies arrive faster than expected—known as a precipitous birth. While this can feel overwhelming, there are ways to slow your baby's descent and protect your perineum.

If you feel the "ring of fire" (a burning sensation as the baby crowns), try quick, choppy breaths—imagine blowing out candles or saying "hehehe" in rapid succession. This type of breathing prompts small, short contractions in the pelvic floor, which can slow the baby's descent and give your tissues time to stretch.

Your body often knows what to do instinctively. If you feel the urge to bring your legs closer together or place your hands on your pelvic floor to slow things down, trust that this is your body's wisdom guiding you.

Perineal Massage: Steps and Tips

Here's a practical guide to starting perineal massage:

Steps:

1. Wash your hands and trim your thumbnails. Set a timer for 5 minutes.

2. Find a comfortable position (e.g., sitting propped up, squatting against a wall, or raising one leg on a stool).

3. Place one thumb about 1–1.5 inches inside your vagina, pressing gently toward your tailbone. Observe what you feel.

4. Practice slow belly breaths, focusing on releasing tension in any tender areas.

5. Gently stretch the tissue between 3 o'clock and 9 o'clock using sweeping motions.

Lubricant Options: Use high-quality, organic products such as:

- Water-soluble lubricant
- Coconut oil
- Vitamin E oil

Partner Support: By week 35, you may find it difficult to reach certain areas. A partner can help by following the same instructions, using their lubricated index finger and focusing on gentle, U-shaped motions. Communication and relaxation are key to making this a positive experience.

Gentleness and preparation are my allies. I trust my body and its ability to lengthen and release.

Chapter 17
Birth Coaching with Pelvic PTs/OTs

PELVIC THERAPY IS NOT just for people who have problems—it's about preventing them. Over the years, my practice has evolved beyond simply treating symptoms to proactively preparing women for birth, both physically and emotionally. Whether it's a first birth or a third, each experience is unique, and every woman deserves to feel ready—not just hopeful that things will go smoothly.

We can only learn so much from books, online courses, and even traditional birth classes. A personalized, in-person assessment reveals exactly what an individual needs in their prenatal journey. Many women assume they will receive this level of preparation from their OBGYN or midwife, but prenatal medical visits have a different purpose. Providers are monitoring the baby's growth, checking the mother's health, and screening for complications like preterm labor or preeclampsia. They have limited time for deeper education on labor preparation and physical readiness.

I recently spoke with a patient who had invested time and money in a six-week birth class, only to finish feeling completely unprepared. She learned about the stages of labor but not how to breathe in a way that connects to her pelvic floor. She wasn't taught about birth positions that optimize space in the pelvis or how to protect her perineum. These are critical elements that can make a real difference in labor and recovery.

That's where pelvic therapy steps in. Each session is tailored to the individual—whether it's addressing existing pain, fitting for lumbar or pelvic support braces, or modifying exercise routines to keep movement safe and effective. We also discuss nutrition and supplements, making sure they are getting what their body needs. It's a fully customized approach, helping women feel not only physically prepared but also confident in their body's ability to give birth.

One of my clients shared her experience after working with us:

"I have learned so much from Buffy. After I had a bad experience with my first birth, I went to Pinnacle. Buffy gave me so many tips and truly made it possible for me to avoid tearing and have natural births with my last two children. She is personable and knowledgeable. I truly cannot say enough great things. Using a pelvic floor therapist before and after birth has truly made my recovery time less."

Another incredible benefit of working with a pelvic PT before birth is the continuity of care postpartum. As unpredictable as birth can be, knowing you already have a trusted provider ready to support your recovery is invaluable. Those who have learned to connect with their core and breath before labor often transition more smoothly into postpartum healing. Even in the early days of holding their baby, they have the awareness to gently reconnect with their core, laying the foundation for a strong recovery.

What Birth Coaching with a Pelvic PT or OT typically Includes:

- Full-body and core/pelvic floor assessment

- Screening for any pelvic issues that may influence labor and treating them

- Teaching breath connection to the core for labor and faster postpartum recovery

- Hands-on work to address joint, muscle and soft tissue restrictions, keeping the body as mobile and comfortable as possible

- Guidance on pain management strategies, partner support, and nervous system regulation to reduce tension and pain perception

- A customized plan to feel empowered and truly ready for birth

We typically see clients in the early second trimester for a screening and initial guidance, then shift to birth preparation by 34–35 weeks. Some women only need two sessions, while others benefit from eight or more, depending on their needs. No matter where they are in their journey, the goal remains the same: to help them step into birth with confidence, knowledge, and a deep trust in their body.

My preparation team is there to guide, support, and empower me every step of the way.

Chapter 18
Back and Belly Support
Taping vs Bracing

During pregnancy, there comes a time when our belly feels quite large, and we might experience aches in our back, pelvis, or abdomen. Support braces can be incredibly helpful in reducing discomfort during this stage.

Amidst the demanding pregnancy journey, there's no need to endure unnecessary misery when simple solutions can make a significant difference. My suggestion? Consider belly taping with kinesiology tape or utilizing lumbar and pelvic supports. These options are straightforward and budget-friendly.

Belly Taping

Us pelvic therapists use kinesiology tape for pregnant belly support. It is usually not necessary till at least week 30. One thing to note is that belly taping requires a longer length of tape than is found with rolls with pre-cut strips found in stores and most sold online. We buy large rolls without perforated strips so that we can apply a length of kinesiology tape from one hip bone to the opposite lower rib to the side of the belly. This tape can stay on for up to 5 days at a time.

Many women like the support that belly taping provides without feeling lower belly compression as is found with a lumbar support.

Note that some of us have more sensitive skin and we can only tolerate the tape for a day before our skin feels itchy or irritated.

Maternity Lumbar Support Braces

A simple lumbar support brace can create a lot of relief for low back pain and even some reduction in round ligament strain/pain. Lumbar support braces are best for when we are on our feet as they will feel like they are digging in our lower belly as soon as we sit down. Trust me, you will want to take the brace off as soon as you sit down. This doesn't mean the brace is useless... it's just most helpful when we have to be on our feet.

Look for a simple maternity lumbar support online that is around $20-$30. Even better, if purchased from a place with a good return policy so you can return it if it does not provide you with some relief.

Chapter 19
Recommended Actions Steps: Third Trimester Through Birth

CREATING SMALL, CONSISTENT HABITS now will prepare your body for labor and make the birth process smoother. These steps are simple and easy to integrate into your daily routine. Remember, the goal isn't perfection—it's progress!

Here's what to focus on:

- **Daily Belly Breathing:** Spend 5–10 minutes practicing belly breathing in different postures. *Habit Stack:* Try this while lying in bed, sitting on the couch, or during a quiet moment after meals.

- **Down Dog or Hands and Knees Stretch:** Add these positions to your daily movement routine to support optimal baby positioning and pelvic mobility.

- **Pelvic Floor Connection:** On your *inhale,* gently bulge your pelvic floor as you breathe in. *Tip:* Try this while lying on your side and place the fingers of your top hand just inside your top sit bone (ischial tuberosity) to feel for movement. Use a clean finger or wand (with lubricant, if needed) if you'd like to assess more deeply.

- **Explore Relaxing Birth Postures:** Experiment with labor positions like side-lying, hands and knees, or using a birth stool. Which ones feel the most supportive and relaxing to you? Practice connecting your breath to your pelvic floor in these positions.

- **Relax Your Jaw:** Check in with your jaw periodically during the day. Is it clenched? Use a slow, 4-count exhale to release tension in your jaw and face.

Consistency Over Perfection

Take it one step at a time—each small action is a step toward feeling confident and prepared. If you miss a day, don't worry! Simply pick up where you left off. The key is to create habits that fit into your rhythm and feel achievable for you.

Practice doesn't make perfect—it makes progress. Every small step matters.

Preparation creates confidence and
confidence creates ease.

What steps are you taking to feel prepared and empowered for your birth experience?

Your preparation is unique to you.

What birth positions or techniques feel most natural or appealing to you?

Turning reflection into action can help you move forward with confidence.

What is one thing you can do this week to connect with your pelvic floor, breath, or core?

How can you involve your birth partner or support team in your preparation?

SECTION III: Labor Support

THINKING ABOUT THE MOMENT your labor begins can bring a mix of emotions—excitement, anticipation, and sometimes a touch of nervousness or anxiety. It's completely natural to feel this way as you prepare for such an incredible, life-changing event. This section is designed to guide you through both the physical and mental aspects of preparing for birth, helping you feel grounded and empowered as the big day approaches.

From creating a calming birth environment to exploring tools like birth balls, rebozos, and affirmations, we'll cover everything you need to feel supported. You'll find practical checklists, journal prompts, and actionable tips to organize your thoughts and ensure you're ready for whatever path your birth takes. By the time you've worked through this section, you'll feel more prepared, more confident, and genuinely excited for the beautiful journey ahead.

Chapter 20
Your Birth Environment

CREATING AN OPTIMAL BIRTH environment is essential for setting the tone for labor, helping you feel in control, and ensuring you are relaxed and comfortable, even if you are delivering in a hospital. The birth environment includes your home, where labor begins, and the birth center or hospital where you may transition. Simple adjustments to the environment can make a significant difference in your birthing experience by engaging all your senses.

Here are some key elements to consider for creating your ideal birth environment:

- **Lighting**:
  - Dim the lights to create a soothing atmosphere.
  - Use battery-operated candles or fairy lights for a warm, soft glow.
  - Consider an eye mask or dark cloth to block out harsh hospital lighting if needed.

- **Aromatherapy**:
  - Incorporate calming or grounding essential oils like lavender for relaxation or citrus scents for energy and upliftment.

- Use a portable diffuser, place a few drops in your palm, or put a few drops on a cotton ball to smell. A cotton ball is easy to remove if you find the scent unhelpful.

- Bring essential oils that you enjoy and that have a grounding or calming effect on you.

- **Sounds and Music**:

  - Prepare a playlist of your favorite calming music, nature sounds, or any audio that brings you comfort and joy.

  - Use a portable speaker or your smartphone to play music softly in the background.

  - Consider guided meditations or affirmations to help maintain a positive and focused mindset.

- **Visuals**:

  - Bring photos or images that make you feel happy and relaxed.

  - Consider a vision board with positive affirmations and birth goals.

  - Choose a focal point in the room that you can concentrate on during contractions.

- **Comfort Items**:

  - Bring items from home that provide comfort, such as your favorite pillow or blanket.

- Consider using a birthing ball, peanut ball, or other comfort aids that help with positioning and movement.

- **Temperature**:

  - Adjust the room temperature to a comfortable level for you.

  - Bring a portable fan or cooling cloths to help regulate your temperature.

- **Hydration and Snacks**:

  - Keep a water bottle within reach to stay hydrated.

  - Have light, healthy snacks available to maintain your energy levels during labor.

- **Support Team**:

  - Ensure your birthing partner and support team are aware of your preferences and birth environment goals.

  - Communicate openly with your healthcare providers about any specific requests or adjustments you need for comfort.

By thoughtfully preparing your birth environment, you can create a space that supports a positive, empowering, and comfortable birthing experience. Taking control of these elements helps you feel more relaxed and in charge, which can contribute to a smoother labor and delivery process.

A calm birth space isn't about having every comfort or recreating a spa. It's about small, intentional choices that help me feel safe, supported, and at ease—wherever I birth.

Chapter 21
Guiding Each Labor Stage: Goals and Partner Support

Stage 1: Early Labor

THE FIRST STAGE OF labor is the initial stage of the birthing process, which includes the onset of uterine contractions that help the cervix to gradually open up or dilate. This stage is divided into two sub-stages: the early or latent stage and the active stage. During the early stage, the cervix dilates from 0 to around 3-4 centimeters. This can take several hours or even days, and contractions may be irregular and mild to moderate in strength. In the active stage, which typically lasts from 3-8 hours, the cervix continues to dilate from 4 to 10 centimeters. Contractions become stronger, longer, and closer together, and the baby starts to descend into the birth canal. The first stage of labor ends once the cervix is fully dilated, and the woman is ready to push the baby out during the second stage.

Goals during the first stage of labor:

- During the initial stage of labor, a key objective is to prepare for the active labor stage. This involves remaining active (gently moving around, changing positions), practicing relaxation methods, and conserving energy. It is essential for the expectant mother to maintain her strength and endurance by eating nourishing foods and hydrating well. Adrenal cocktails can be a great help for both hydration and energy support.

- Creating a comforting and secure environment is vital at this stage. This may involve keeping the room softly lit, playing calming music, and utilizing aromatherapy or massage for relaxation. The mother-to-be should feel supported and motivated by her birthing team, which may include her partner or a doula if she has one.

- Effectively managing pain and discomfort is another significant aim during this stage of labor. Techniques like breathing (or zen breathing as it is sometimes called), visualization, and other relaxation methods can assist in coping with contractions. Pain relief options, including medication, could also be considered based on individual circumstances and preferences.Partner Tips:

Supporting Your Partner During Early Labor

This is your time to step up and be your partner's biggest cheerleader. Early labor is often the longest part of the process, so your calm, steady presence can make a world of difference. Here are some simple ways to help during this stage:

Stay Calm and Reassuring: Your energy sets the tone. If you're calm, it'll help your partner feel calmer too. Offer encouraging words like, *"You're doing great,"* or just be there quietly so they know you've got their back. Even holding their hand can speak volumes.

Bring the Comfort: Think about what makes your partner feel relaxed and try to make it happen. Adjust the lights, grab a cozy blanket, or turn on some music they love. A back rub, a foot massage, or just gently rubbing their shoulders can work wonders when things get intense. Apply pressure to both sides of their pelvis with your hands or use a sarong wrapped low around their hips.

Keep Them Hydrated and Fed: Labor is a marathon, and staying hydrated and nourished is key. Offer water, ice chips, or small snacks if they're up for it (check with the care team first). Don't push—sometimes all they'll want is a sip here or there.

Encourage Movement and Watch the Clock: If your partner's up for it, help them move around. Walking, swaying, or even leaning forward on a birth ball can help keep labor progressing. Think of birth as a dance between mother and baby. Changing positions regularly helps them work together to make progress. Encourage and support them in shifting their positioning every 20-30 minutes.

Offer Distractions: Early labor can feel like a long wait. Help pass the time by watching a favorite show together, having a lighthearted chat, or playing some music they enjoy. Sometimes, just being there and sharing the moment is the best distraction of all.

Transition

The transition stage of labor stands out as the most intense and demanding part of the birthing process. It signifies the final segment of the initial labor stage, marked by powerful and frequent contractions that facilitate the cervix expanding from 8 to 10 centimeters.

In these crucial moments, many of us may feel overwhelmed and uncertain, thinking "we don't got this" which often signals to our birth team that the end is near. Typically lasting from 30 minutes to 2 hours, this stage showcases stronger, longer, and closer contractions, along with heightened pressure and discomfort in the lower back and pelvis for the mother. As the baby progresses through the birth canal, the mother may feel the urge to push.

Goals For Transition:

- Maintaining focus and composure, managing pain, and preparing for childbirth. Deep and slow breathing is essential to stay focused and alleviate pain. All the breathing exercises and preparation will prove invaluable here!

- Staying hydrated and well-rested is another priority, as fatigue and dehydration can heighten the challenges of the transition stage. Electrolyte drinks or an Adrenal Cocktail are highly recommended throughout labor, especially during this critical stage. Ultimately, the transition stage aims to ensure a safe and successful progression to the pushing stage for both mother and baby.

Supporting Your Partner During the Transition stage

The transition stage is often the most intense and challenging part of labor. This is your moment to really shine as the ultimate support system. Stay calm, be present, and remember: your steady presence can make all the difference. Here's how to help during this critical time:

Be Attentive and Supportive: This is where your partner needs you the most. Transition can feel overwhelming, so be ready with words of encouragement like, *"You're so strong—I'm in awe of you,"* or *"You're almost there; you've got this."* Pay close attention to their cues and be ready to adjust as needed.

Encourage Deep Breathing: Help your partner focus on slow, deep breaths to manage the intensity of the contractions. If they start to feel panicked or lose rhythm, gently guide them back with a steady voice: *"Breathe in deeply... now slowly let it out."* Breathing together can create a sense of connection and calm.

Stay Fully Present: Put your phone away, clear your mind, and give your full attention. Listen actively to what your partner needs, whether it's water, a position change, or simply a reassuring touch. Even if they're not saying much, stay in tune with their body language.

Offer Physical Support: This is the time to put your practice into action. Apply hip pressure, rub their back, or offer your hands for them to hold. If they want to change positions, be ready to help them adjust safely. If you're unsure what they need, just ask: *"Would this feel good, or do you want to try something else?"*

Remind Them of the End Goal: When the contractions are at their most intense, remind your partner of what's on the other side: *"Each wave is bringing us closer to meeting our baby."* Acknowledge their strength and progress with heartfelt words like, *"Look how far you've come—you're incredible."*

This is the stage where your calm, confident energy can help your partner feel grounded and supported. Keep your focus on them, and remember, you're a team in this together.

Stage 2: Pushing Stage

The second stage of labor is the stage of childbirth where the baby comes earthside. It begins when the cervix is fully dilated (open) and ends when the baby is born. This stage can take anywhere from a few minutes to a few hours, depending on various factors such as the size of the baby, the position of the baby, and the strength of the mother's contractions. During this stage, the mother will feel a strong urge to push as the baby moves down the birth canal. The healthcare provider will monitor the baby's progress and may assist with the delivery if necessary. After the baby is born, the umbilical cord is cut, and the body moves into the third stage of labor, when the placenta is delivered and the birth process is completed.

Goals for the mother during the pushing stage of labor:

- **To effectively push the baby down the birth canal:** we need to use our abdominal muscles to push the baby through the birth canal and out.

- We want to be in postures that allow our baby to pass through our pelvic outlet which should be with hips more neutral or slightly internally rotated and allow our tailbone to be untucked.

- **To breathe through contractions:** Contractions can be intense during the pushing stage, and it is important for you to *breathe* through them! Ideally, we should **inhale** to **prepare,** and **exhale** while we **push.** Birth providers have been guiding women to sustain a prolonged breath hold while pushing for many years... this is physiologically *not* ideal. This causes us to reflexively tense our pelvic floor muscles which can slow down delivery, increase chance of perineal tearing, and reduce oxygen to mom and baby. Only in a pinch, or if things are just not working to breathe with our efforts should we resort to breath holds.

- **Move through our contractions:** holding our body like it is a statue is not the goal here. Helping to move through and release the intensity of what we are feeling requires movement. This can be as little as shifting our hips slightly or untucking our tailbone as we work to inhale and release tension.

- **To communicate with the birth team:** we need to communicate our needs and our birth team can provide guidance, support, and pain relief measures if necessary.

- **To remain calm and focused:** The pushing stage can be physically and emotionally demanding. We should try to remain calm and focused, and draw strength from our support team. *This is where our affirmations can be of help*. Focus on your baby and getting to see their beautiful face for the first time!

Overall, the goals for the mother during the pushing stage of labor are to push the baby down the birth canal, breathe through contractions, communicate with their support team and healthcare provider, and remain calm and focused.

Supporting Your Partner During the Pushing Stage

The pushing stage marks the final stretch of labor—an exciting but intense time for your partner. Your role here is to stay calm, steady, and supportive as they work through this monumental effort. This is where teamwork and encouragement matter most. Here's how you can help:

Be Attentive and Supportive: This is it—the finish line is in sight! Let your partner know how incredible they are with words of encouragement like, *"You're so close to meeting our baby,"* or *"You're doing an amazing job; I'm so proud of you."* Stay present and responsive to their needs, whether it's holding their hand or just being a steady presence by their side.

Encourage Breathing with the Push: Help your partner stay connected to their breath during this stage. Remind them to take a deep inhale before bearing down and to release tension as they exhale. If they're struggling, guide them gently: *"Take a deep breath in, and now let's push together on the next contraction."*

Stay Fully Present: Be completely engaged in the moment. Watch for cues from your partner and respond with empathy and attentiveness. Your calm presence can make them feel secure and supported during this demanding stage.

Offer Physical Support: Provide physical support however it's needed. This might mean giving compression to both sides of their pelvis with your hands or using a sarong wrapped around them, holding their hand, rubbing their shoulders, or helping them stabilize in a comfortable birthing position. If they're pushing in an upright position, you might even physically support their weight if needed. Always check in: *"Do you want to try a different position?"* or *"Does this feel okay?"*

Remind Them of the End Goal: Keep the focus on the joy and reward that lies ahead: *"You're doing it—we're about to meet our baby!"* Affirm their strength and capabilities with genuine statements like, *"You've worked so hard to get here, and I know you can do this."*

The pushing stage is a momentous and emotional time. Your encouragement, presence, and physical support will make all the difference in helping your partner feel strong, capable, and ready to meet your baby.

Partner Support
Checklist

Early Labor

- Stay Calm and Reassuring:
  - Your energy sets the tone. Offer encouraging words like, "You're doing great" or just hold their hand to show support.
  - Stay calm to help your partner feel calmer too.
- Bring the Comfort:
  - Adjust lights, provide cozy blankets, or play relaxing music.
  - Use any support tools you have (birth comb, TENS unit for back, cupping tools), apply pelvic pressure with your hands or sarong.
- Keep Them Hydrated and Fed:
  - Offer small sips of water, ice chips, or light snacks if allowed.
- Encourage Movement:
  - Help them change positions every 20-30 minutes (e.g., walking, swaying, leaning on a birth ball or CUB).
- Offer Distractions:
  - Watch a show, chat, or play their favorite music to help pass the time.

Transition

- Be Attentive and Supportive:
  - Provide encouragement: "You're so strong" or "You're almost there."
  - Pay attention to their cues and adjust support as needed.
- Encourage Deep Breathing:
  - Gently guide them with slow, deep breaths: "Breathe in deeply... and slowly let it out."
  - Breathe together to create connection and calm.
- Stay Fully Present:
  - Put distractions away and focus on what they need (e.g., water, position changes, reassurance).

Partner Support
Checklist

Transition (continued)

- Offer Physical Support:
  - Apply hip pressure, rub their back, or help them move into new positions.
  - Check in: "Does this feel good, or would you like to try something else?"
- Remind Them of the End Goal:
  - Keep them focused on the baby: "Each wave is bringing us closer to meeting our baby."
  - Affirm their progress: "Look how far you've come—you're amazing."

Pushing Stage

- Be Attentive and Encouraging:
  - Offer affirmations: "You're so close to meeting our baby" or "You're doing an incredible job."
- Encourage Breathing with the Push:
  - Remind them to take a deep breath in before, and blow out to push. Note: their tailbone should be more untucked with effective pushing and a good sign that their pelvic floor is not tensing up.
- Stay Fully Present:
  - Be engaged and attentive. Respond to their cues with empathy and support.
- Offer Physical Support:
  - Provide pelvic compression, rub their shoulders, or stabilize them in a birthing position.
  - Check in: "Do you want to try a different position?" or "Does this feel okay?"
- Remind Them of the End Goal:
  - Focus on the reward: "You're doing it, we're about to meet our baby!"
  - Acknowledge their strength: "You're doing amazing."

Chapter 22
Labor Support Tools and Techniques

When it comes to supporting us mentally and physically during our labor, there are *many* options. We will go through many of these options and you can decide which sound most appealing to you are which ones you would like to try with your support person. This is *definitely* the part of the book you want them to read *with* you!

Techniques we will review include:

- Rebozo wrap

- Dynamic Cupping to the middle and lower back

- Deep pressure strokes upper back to hips

- Pelvic Hug/ Compression (can use the wrap)

- TENS unit for low back or belly

Rebozo

The Rebozo is a traditional Mexican shawl or scarf that has been used for centuries as a versatile tool in various aspects of Mexican culture and daily life. In recent years, it has gained popularity in the context of childbirth and has become a valuable tool for providing support and comfort to women during labor.

During childbirth, the Rebozo is used by trained birth attendants, midwives, or doulas to support and assist women through various stages of labor. Partners can learn some of these techniques as well which is where your partner comes in!

Here are some ways the Rebozo is used to support women in childbirth:

- **Pain relief and relaxation**: The Rebozo can be used to gently wrap around the woman's body to create counter-pressure and provide relief from pain during contractions. The even pressure and warmth can help the mother to relax and cope with the intensity of labor.

- **Positioning:** The Rebozo can be used to help the mother get into different positions that may aid in labor progress and provide comfort. For instance, it can be used to support the mother in a squatting position, on hands and knees, or in a supported side-lying position.

- **Pelvic rocking**: The Rebozo can be employed to facilitate gentle pelvic rocking or swaying, which can help the baby find an optimal position for birth and encourage progress in the labor process.

- **Assistance during pushing**: The Rebozo can be utilized to provide support as the mother pushes during the second stage of labor. It can be held by the birth attendant to provide stability and resistance for the mother to push against.

Note: You can use a large sarong or a traditional Rebozo (traditional from Mexico).

Rebozo Techniques

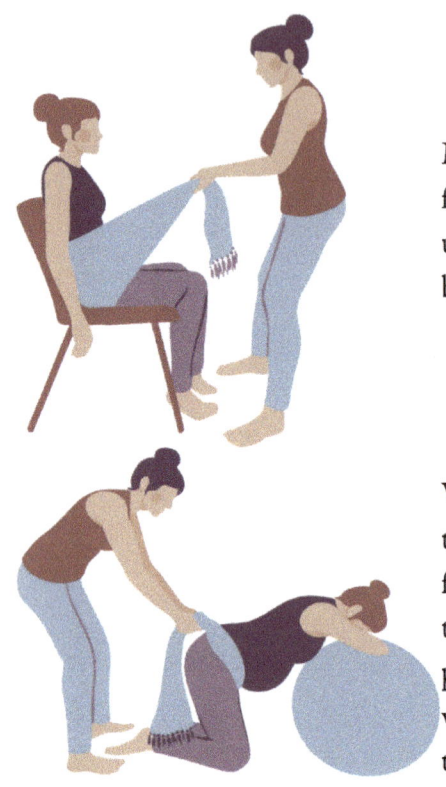

Seated Hip/Pelvic Pressure:
Mom is sitting on wrap and partner facing each other. Partner pulls in upward diagonal direction for low back relief.

Pelvic Counter Pressure:
Wrap a sarong or rebozo low around the birthing mom's hips. Cross the fabric behind her back and gently pull to compress the hips to the level of pressure she prefers. Twist the the wrap to secure the tension and hold the twist to maintain steady counter pressure.

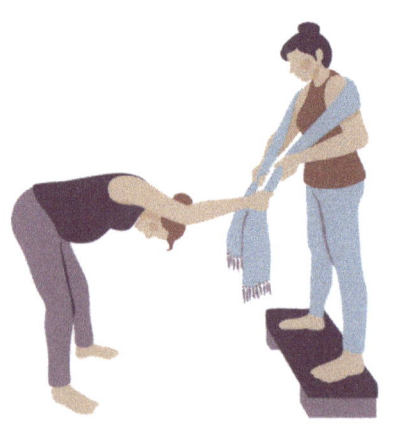

Forward Fold:
Drape the wrap over the partner's shoulders like a shawl. The birthing mom holds one end of the fabric in each hand and folds forward from the hips, keeping a flat back and soft knees. She may gently sway side to side or bend and straighten her knees for comfort and release.

Rebozo Techniques

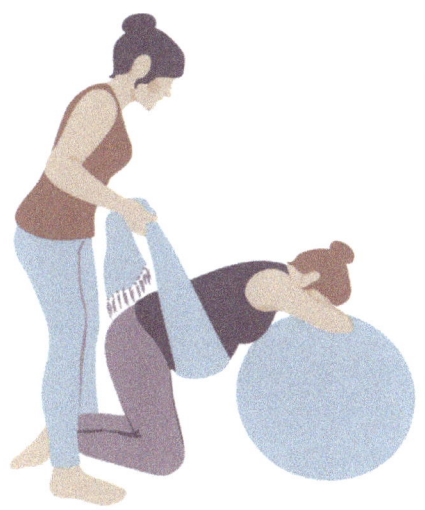

Hands and Knees Belly Sifting:
Place the wrap under the belly while the birthing mom is on hands and knees. The partner gently lifts the fabric to cradle the belly, then softly sifts or jiggles the wrap to release tension and provide soothing support through the belly and low back.

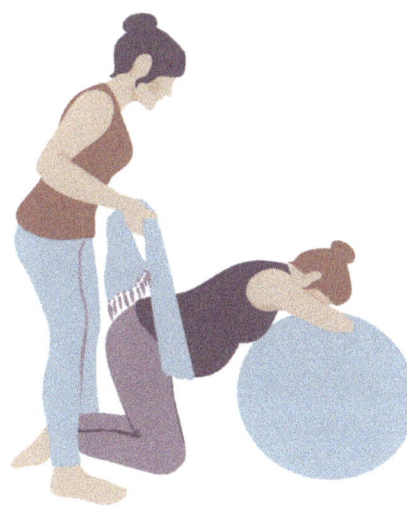

Hands and Knees Hip Sifting:
Place the wrap under the hips and gather the fabric at each side. The partner gently wiggles or lifts one side at a time to create a rhythmic, soothing motion through the hips.

Not pictured: The partner may also place the wrap over the top of the hips, holding the fabric at each side and gently pressing down in a soft, jiggling or sifting motion to release tension.

Dynamic Cupping To The Middle and Lower Back

Using a silicone cupping tool has got to be one of my *favorite* techniques to teach a partner! Traditionally, cupping tools are used in Chinese medicine made of glass and suction is created and placed on the body and left there for a period of minutes. With silicone tools, we can create suction and move the cup along the back as long as we have some lotion or balm rubbed onto the skin first.

This provides a lot of increased blood flow and helps with mobilizing and stretching muscle and fascia to relieve all of the ever increasing low back tension that us pregnant women develop as our body changes.

When to use this technique:

- *During Pregnancy* (especially by week 30)

- *During Labor*

- *Postpartum* (the back doesn't magically stop being tense and cupping the low back can help with allowing our abdominals to come back together).

What is needed: All that is needed is a good muscle balm or lotion that has some shea butter or oil base that doesn't quickly get absorbed by the skin and a 2 to 2.5-inch silicon cupping tool you can purchase online.

How to do it:

1. Apply the muscle balm to the skin.

2. Press thumb into the top of the silicon cup to apply pressure to

the back to create a suction. Place the cup onto the skin to create a seal.

3. Then glide the cup slowly over the back. The person doing the cupping should rely on their pregnant partner for feedback on how much suction and what areas feel good to her.

Most people find that about 10 minutes of cupping at a time feels great.

Deep Pressure Strokes from Head to Hips

While mom is seated and leaning over while supported by a bed, ball, or back of chair, you can apply a firm pressure with the heels of your hands in a downward direction starting at her upper back and moving down and then outward toward her hips. This firm pressure feels really good to her tense low back and will feel soothing and can act as a great counter pressure for contractions.

It is also known that firm pressure stroked from head to tail calms the nervous system, which is ideal in labor. This can be done for as long as you would like or as long as it feels good to you.

Pelvic Compression/Hug

It can be very relieving to have your hips compressed from both sides during a contraction. Your partner can apply this compression with their elbows held out wide to either side and applying a force with their hands.

This can also be created with the Rebozo or wrap. Drape the middle of the wrap below your belly and then crossed at your low back. You can choose how much compression you like, and then our partner can lock it out by twisting the wrap once the desired tension is created. All that needs to be done at this point is hold onto the twisted fabric, making it a technique that your partner can sustain for as long as you need as it doesn't not require a lot of work or effort. We found this to be a welcome technique for a couple that the birth partner had had an arm injury and could not use one hand very easily. He was relieved that he could be of help in this capacity.

This technique can be applied with mom in multiple positions including hands and knees, sitting, or side lying... as long as we have access to your back. The only difference in side lying is that we would just apply pressure to the top hip. With the need to be moving positions every 20-30 minutes during labor to help things to progress, this compression technique should probably also be limited to 20 minutes as well. You can try other postures and come back to this technique again later.

TENS Unit for Low Back or Belly

A TENS (Transcutaneous Electrical Nerve Stimulation) unit is a small, portable device that delivers mild electrical impulses through electrodes placed on the skin. It is commonly used for pain relief in various conditions, including during labor. When used correctly, a TENS unit can be a non-invasive and drug-free method to help manage labor pain. Here's how it can be used for a laboring woman:

The TENS unit comes with sticky electrode pads that are placed strategically on the laboring woman's back. The most common placement is along the lower back, on either side of the spine. The positioning may vary depending on the woman's individual needs and where she feels the most pain during contractions.

- **Adjustable settings**: The TENS unit allows for adjusting the intensity and frequency of the electrical impulses. You can control these settings during contractions to find the most comfortable level of stimulation for you.

- **Gate control theory**: The TENS unit works on the principle of the gate control theory of pain. The electrical impulses stimulate the nerves and interfere with the transmission of pain signals to the brain, essentially "closing the gate" and reducing the perception of pain.

TENS can be used in combination with other non-invasive pain relieving strategies. Fortunately, a TENS unit can be purchased online for around thirty dollars.

TENS Unit For Low Back

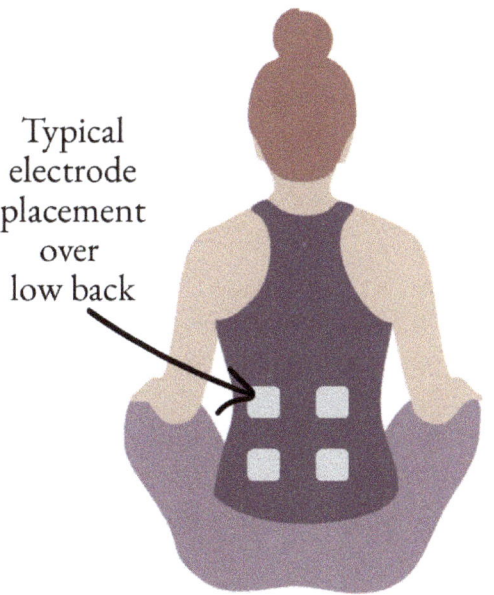

Typical electrode placement over low back

*Every tool I use is a sign of
wisdom and resourcefulness.*

Chapter 23
The Best Birthing Positions For The Pushing Phase

The best positions for a vaginal childbirth can vary depending on the individual. What is important is that we are in positions that:

- You feel like you can push effectively and allow your pelvic floor muscles to relax

- your pelvis is able to move and widen in the pelvic outlet (ideally. not on our back, hips more neutral or internally rotated).

- You feel SUPPORTED and comfortable.

It's important to keep in mind that each woman's experience is unique, and what works well for one individual may not be the best option for another. Additionally, the labor process is dynamic, and changing positions during labor every 20-30 minutes is ideal. Some positions may be more suitable for certain stages of labor than others. It's crucial for your birthing team to be supportive and flexible in assisting you in finding the most comfortable and effective positions for you as well as keep an eye on the clock and help you move into a different position every 30 minutes to help your labor progress well.

Birth Positions

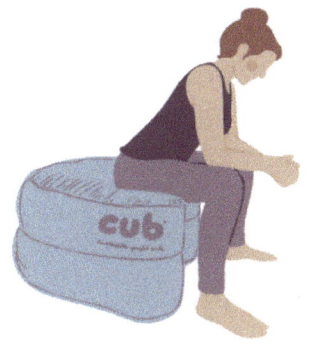

Squatting positions:

Deep squat: This position widens the pelvic outlet, allowing more room for the baby to descend. It can be done with support from a partner or a squatting bar. Note: most Westerners are not used to being in a deep squat for prolonged times. This posture is not ideal if you are not used to being in a squat for more than a few minutes comfortably.

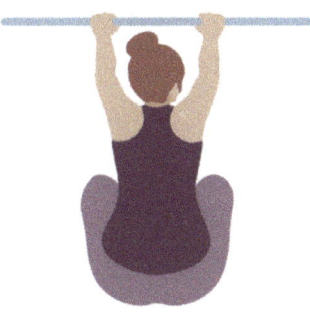

Supported squat: Squatting with the support of a doula, partner, squatting bar, or birthing stool can be much less strenuous, and you can likely be in this posture for longer periods.

Hands and Knees:

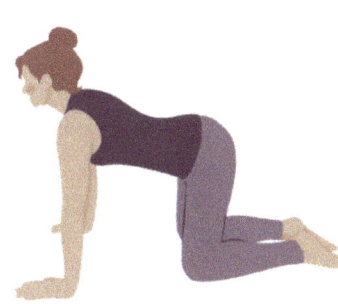

Being on hands and knees can relieve pressure on the back and help rotate a baby in a posterior position (facing the mother's abdomen) to an anterior position (facing the mother's back).

This position is also associated with the Gaskin Maneuver (named after Ina May Gaskin). When a baby's head emerges but the shoulders are "stuck". Instead of an invasive technique being used such as an episiotomy, the mother is assisted into hands and knees posture to allow her pelvis to open further and birth her baby without injury to her body.

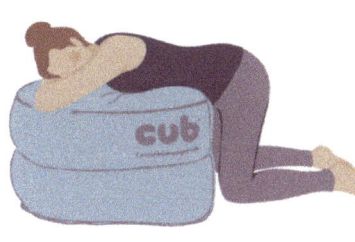

Birth Positions

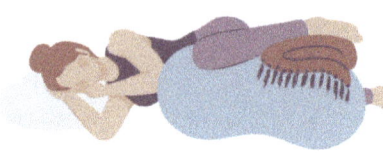

Side-lying positions:
Lying on one side with knees bent: This position can be comfortable during early labor and provides a restful option between contractions. Many women find that they can effectively push and allow their pelvic floor muscles to release well in side lying.

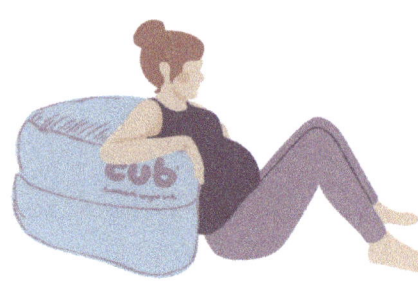

Semi-Reclining Positions:
Leaning back on a birth ball, CUB or reclined in a hospital bed: These positions can provide support while still allowing gravity to aid in the downward movement of baby.

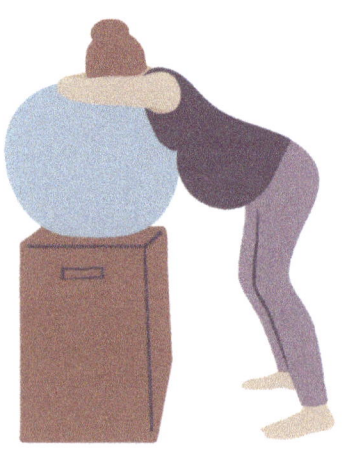

Upright positions:
Standing: Standing and swaying or rocking can help encourage the baby's downward movement and progress labor.

Leaning forward: Leaning on a counter, table, or a birthing ball can take pressure off the back and pelvis and open up the pelvic outlet.

Chapter 24

Jaw, Neck, and Shoulder Tension Relieving Strategies

Before and During Birth

Jaw and neck tension can have significant effects on childbirth, and the relationship between these areas of the body and the birthing process is often referred to as the "jaw-neck connection." Here's how jaw and neck tension can influence childbirth:

- **Connection with the pelvic floor**: The jaw and pelvic floor are interconnected through a fascial network known as the deep front line. Tension in the jaw and neck can be mirrored in the pelvic floor muscles, leading to tightness and potential restrictions. During childbirth, relaxed and supple pelvic floor muscles are essential for the baby's descent through the birth canal. Jaw and neck tension can indirectly hinder the release and relaxation of the pelvic floor muscles, making it more challenging for the baby to move down during labor.

- **Autonomic Nervous System Response and Psychological Impact:** Tension in the jaw and neck can trigger stress responses in the autonomic nervous system, specifically activating the sympathetic nervous system responsible for the "fight or flight" response. This activation leads to an increased release of stress hormones like cortisol and adrenaline, which can interfere with the production of oxytocin, the hormone essential for promoting labor contractions. Insufficient oxytocin levels may slow or stall labor progress. Additionally, jaw and neck tension is often linked with anxiety, fear, or a sense of holding back, which can negatively impact the birthing experience. These emotions heighten pain perception and inhibit the release of endorphins, the body's natural pain-relieving hormones.

- **Impact on Breathing:** Jaw and neck tension can significantly affect breathing patterns during labor. When these areas are tense, shallow and restricted breathing becomes common, reducing oxygen levels and causing the body to perceive stress. Proper breathing is essential during childbirth as it helps oxygenate the mother and baby and keeps the mother calm and relaxed, facilitating a smoother birthing process.

Addressing jaw and neck tension before and during childbirth can be beneficial for a smoother and more positive birthing experience.

Techniques that can help alleviate tension in these areas include:

- Relaxation techniques: Practicing relaxation exercises, such as deep breathing, mindfulness, and progressive muscle relaxation, can help reduce overall tension in the body, including the jaw and neck.

- Bodywork and massage: Receiving gentle bodywork or massage focused on the neck, shoulders, and jaw can release tension and promote relaxation.

- Conscious jaw and neck relaxation: During labor, being aware of and consciously relaxing the jaw and neck can help break the tension-stress cycle and support a more relaxed state of being.

- Overall, maintaining relaxation and reducing tension in the jaw and neck can positively influence the physiological and psychological aspects of childbirth, contributing to a more comfortable and efficient labor process.

To Work On Now:

- Minimize forward head postures

- Use head rests (in car, watching TV, etc)

- Practice Resting Jaw Position (front ½ of tongue gently touching the palate, teeth not touching and lips closed)

- Break up longer stretches of reading, computer time with gentle rotations/wiggles of neck and jaw.

During Labor:

- Good neck support

- Have a partner spot your jaw for tension

- Practicing breathing with a relaxed jaw (Inhale with nose and jaw relaxed, softly blow out for the same amount of time as inhale. For example: Inhale for 4 counts; blow softly for 4 counts.

Chapter 25

Vocalization

Channeling Strength and Releasing Tension in Labor

Vocalization is more than a way to stay calm in labor—it's a way to harness your strength, release resistance, and work with your body as you bring your baby into the world. Sound has the power to ground you, keep the pelvic floor from clenching, and carry the force of your effort in a productive way.

By releasing sound through the throat, we create a natural connection down to the pelvic floor, reminding those muscles to soften rather than fight against contractions. Sometimes this takes the form of deep, low sounds that soothe and relax. At other times, especially in the pushing stage, it can build into what many birth workers call the *"woman's roar"*—a powerful, primal sound that channels your strength and energy into helping your baby descend.

This is your time—there is no need to stay silent or to worry about disturbing others. Let your voice rise and fall with your labor. Whether soft and steady or strong and forceful, vocalization can help you stay grounded, reduce pain, and work with your body rather than against it.

Why Vocalization Helps

- Releases the energy of each contraction, reducing pain and tension.

- Helps the nervous system shift into a calmer, more focused state.

- Prevents pelvic floor muscles from tightening against labor surges, allowing for a smoother birth.

- Channels strength and effort into sound, supporting effective pushing.

- Activates the Throat Chakra (expression) and Root Chakra (grounding and release) to support an open, connected flow from voice to pelvis.

Vocalization Techniques for Labor

Your sounds may shift as labor progresses—sometimes low and soothing, other times strong and powerful. All of it is natural, and all of it can help you work with your body rather than against it.

- Low, Open Sounds: Deep tones like "Ooo" or "Ahh" help relax the jaw and throat, which signals the pelvic floor to release.

- Moaning or Humming: A steady hum or moan can be grounding, helping you ride the rhythm of each contraction.

- Exhaling with Sound: Inhale deeply, then exhale slowly with a sound like "Haaa," letting tension flow downward and out.

- The Woman's Roar: As pushing intensifies, vocalization may rise into a strong, primal roar. This isn't uncontrolled screaming—it's a focused release of strength and energy that channels your power into helping your baby descend.

My voice is a powerful tool—release my energy, calm my body, and guide my baby closer.

Chapter 26
Using Inflatable Devices:

INFLATABLE DEVICES LIKE THE CUB (Comfortable Upright Birth), birth balls, and peanut balls are versatile tools that can support women throughout labor and delivery, helping to promote comfort, encourage optimal fetal positioning, and relieve pain. Here's a look at how each of these tools can be used:

The Comfortable Upright Birth (CUB)

The CUB is an inflatable support designed to help laboring women maintain upright positions. This positioning can be beneficial for both mother and baby and may result in a smoother labor experience. The CUB offers several potential benefits:

- **Improves Positioning**: Upright positions can encourage the baby to move into an optimal position for birth by creating more space in the pelvis, which may help facilitate progress.

- **Shortens Labor**: Research suggests that staying upright can shorten the first stage of labor by up to 50%.

- **Reduces Complications**: Upright positioning with the CUB can reduce the risk of complications such as the need for medically assisted birth, episiotomy, or emergency cesarean section.

- **Relieves Pain**: The CUB can be used during pregnancy and labor to relieve pelvic and lower back discomfort.

Birth Positions with CUB

The CUB (Comfortable Upright Birth) gives you more options to labor in upright, supported positions. Here are three postures many women find helpful. You can adjust the firmness to what feels best for you.

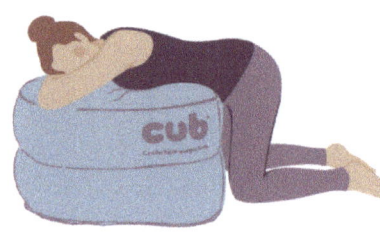

Supported Hands and Knees
Kneel with your belly resting in the CUB's opening and your arms and head supported on top. This position helps relieve back pressure, encourages baby's optimal positioning, and allows your belly to hang naturally for comfort and space.

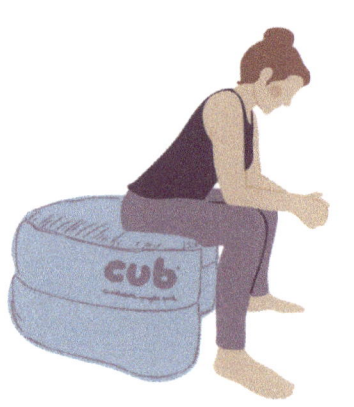

Seated, Leaning Forward
Sit on the CUB with your feet grounded and lean your elbows on your knees. This forward-leaning posture opens the pelvis and allows gentle movement or rocking during contractions. Compared to a birth ball, the CUB offers more stability, helping you feel secure and balanced throughout labor.

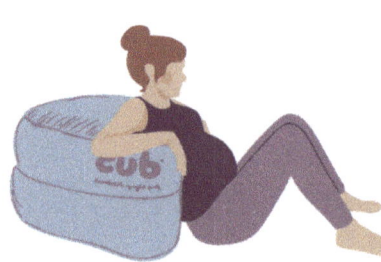

Supported Upright Sitting
Sit upright on the floor or bed with your back supported by the CUB. This position offers rest while staying upright, encourages pelvic opening, and uses gravity to help with laboring down as baby descends.

Birth Balls

Birth balls, also known as birthing or exercise balls, are large, inflatable balls that offer multiple options for comfort, relaxation, and pelvic movement during labor.

- **Comfort and Relaxation**: Sitting, leaning, or kneeling on a birth ball can relieve back pain and promote relaxation through gentle bouncing or rocking.

- **Pelvic Movement and Progress**: The ball allows for free pelvic movement, helping the baby descend into the birth canal. Rocking or rotating on the ball may aid in opening the pelvis and encouraging the baby's optimal positioning.

- **Encouraging Dilation**: Gentle hip circles or rocking on the birth ball can help open and stretch the cervix, potentially assisting with dilation.

Ways to Use the Birth Ball:

1. Sit and gently rock or do hip circles.

2. Place the ball on your bed, lean over it with your arms to either rest with them statically folded over the ball and resting head on arms or roll the ball away and reach arms forward to let your belly relax while releasing back tension.

3. Get on all fours with arms over the ball to release tension in the belly and tailbone while breathing deeply.

4. Lightly bounce on the ball during early labor for additional relief.

Peanut Balls

The peanut ball, a peanut-shaped exercise ball, is ideal for supporting women in side-lying positions during labor.

- **Support in the Side-Lying Position**: Placing a peanut ball between the knees in a side-lying position can be helpful for rest and can facilitate fetal rotation or descent.

- **Promoting Optimal Fetal Positioning**: The shape and placement of the peanut ball create space in the pelvis, encouraging the baby's head to move downward and rotate into a favorable position.

- **Back Pain Relief**: Using the peanut ball behind the back while reclining or seated can provide support and alleviate back pain during labor.

Peanut Ball Birth Positions

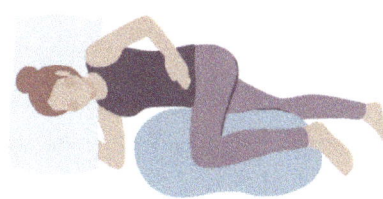

Side-lying
Lying on your side with the bottom leg resting on the bed and the top leg supported by the peanut ball. The top hip and shoulder can be gently rolled forward or back for comfort. Suitable for use in both the 1st and 2nd stages of labor.

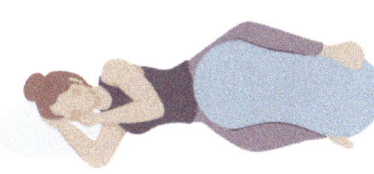

Peanut Ball Between Both Knees
Lying on your side in a curled, fetal-like posture with hips and knees flexed forward. The peanut ball is positioned between both knees for support. Suitable for use in the 1st or 2nd stage of labor.

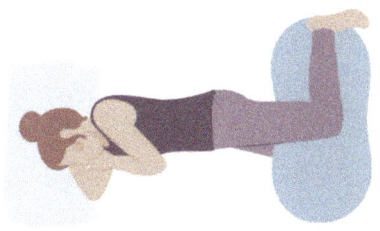

"Flying Cowgirl" (1st Stage)
Lying on your side with the peanut ball positioned between both lower legs. Thighs stay in line with the body while the tailbone is gently tucked under.

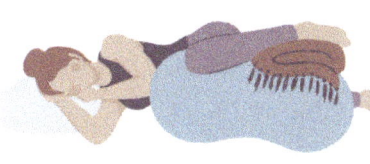

Top Ankle Elevated (2nd Stage)
Lying on your side with the peanut ball placed under the top leg. The ankle is propped higher than the knee, creating gentle internal rotation at the hip to help open the pelvic outlet.

Both the CUB, birth balls, and peanut balls offer laboring women freedom of movement and the ability to explore positions that feel best for them. While many hospitals and birthing centers offer these tools, it's a good idea to check their availability in advance and discuss options with your healthcare provider or birthing team. With the growing popularity of the CUB, I have known of women purchasing one and then selling it to a friend who is also expecting. Experimenting with different positions using the CUB, birth balls, or peanut balls can help you find the most comfortable and effective ways to labor.

Chapter 29
When Is it Time to Push?

BEFORE THE MOTHER BEGINS to push during labor, it is generally preferred for the baby to be in the "0 station" or engaged in the pelvis. The station is a measurement used in obstetrics to describe the position of the baby's presenting part (usually the head) in relation to the maternal pelvis.

Here's a brief explanation of the station scale:

- **Negative Stations (e.g., -1, -2, -3):** The baby's head is above the level of the ischial spines (the bony prominence in the pelvic cavity). This indicates that the baby has not yet descended into the pelvic inlet.

- **0 Station:** The baby's head is at the level of the ischial spines, also known as being engaged. This is the optimal position for the baby before the mother begins to push.

- **Positive Stations (e.g., +1, +2, +3):** The baby's head has passed below the level of the ischial spines and is descending further down the birth canal.

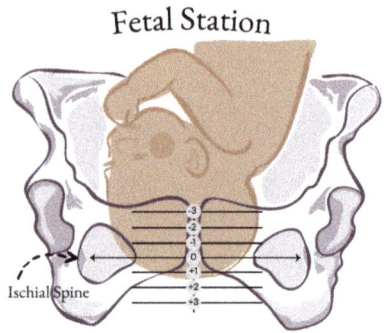

Fetal Station

When the baby is at the 0 station, it means that the head is in the mother's pelvis and is aligned with the ischial spines. This engagement is a positive sign that the baby is well-positioned for birth, and the cervix is usually fully dilated, indicating that the mother can begin pushing during the second stage of labor.

It's important to note that the progression of labor is unique to each individual, and factors such as the mother's pelvic structure, the size and position of the baby, and the strength and effectiveness of contractions can influence the descent of the baby. Healthcare providers closely monitor these factors during labor to determine the optimal time for the mother to begin pushing.

Important Note Regarding Pushing In Childbirth:

*If a mother does **not** have the urge to push and is being asked to do so, they should inquire about the baby's station and dilation level.*

Pushing is most effective when the dilation level is at 10, and the baby is at the zero station. However, in some cases, mothers may be asked to push when they're fully dilated, but the baby hasn't reached the zero station yet.

In such situations, it's appropriate to postpone pushing until the baby has progressed further down in the pelvis. This is known as "laboring down".

Moreover, continuous movement and relaxation techniques can help release muscles around the pelvis, making it easier for the baby to descend further. Remember, "Motion in Lotion!"

Chapter 30
Mindset and Affirmations

THE POWER OF MINDSET and affirmations in preparing for childbirth cannot be overstated. A positive mindset and the use of affirmations can significantly impact a woman's childbirth experience, helping her feel more confident, empowered, and in control.

Additionally, it is in our best interest to learn how to calm our mind and get into a rest-and-digest state regardless of our surroundings... especially when planning a hospital birth. Labors can sometimes stall due to the mother being stressed and anxious as her body will not let the birth progress when not feeling safe. Making time to regularly work on breathing and meditation can help us to build this skill.

How Affirmations Can Support Your Birth

Here are some ways mindset and affirmations can be powerful in childbirth preparation:

- **Reducing fear and anxiety:** Positive affirmations can counteract negative thoughts and fears, promoting a sense of calmness and reducing anxiety about the birthing process.

- **Enhancing confidence:** Affirmations can instill a sense of self-assurance and belief in a woman's ability to birth her baby.

- **Fostering relaxation and focus:** Mindset and affirmations can encourage relaxation during labor, helping to release oxytocin, a hormone vital for effective contractions and labor progress.

- **Shifting perspectives on pain:** Affirmations can help reframe pain as powerful surges bringing your baby closer.

- **Cultivating a positive birth experience:** A positive outlook and the use of affirmations can contribute to a more satisfying birth experience, regardless of how the birth unfolds.

- **Empowering decision-making:** A positive mindset can empower women to advocate for themselves and make informed decisions during labor and birth.

Using Affirmations Effectively

- **Personalize affirmations:** Tailor affirmations to resonate with your specific desires and intentions for childbirth.

- **Use the present tense:** Phrase affirmations as if they are already happening. For example, "I am strong and capable" or "My body knows how to birth my baby."

- **Repeat regularly:** Practice affirmations daily during pregnancy to reinforce positive beliefs.

- **Incorporate them into relaxation techniques:** Use affirmations during meditation, deep breathing exercises, or visualization practices.

- **Surround yourself with positivity:** Create a supportive environment with positive birth stories, affirmations, and encouraging people.

Remember, every birth experience is unique. The goal of affirmations is not to control the outcome but to approach childbirth with a positive and empowered perspective.

Affirmations for Phases of Labor

Early Labor

- My body was made to give birth, and I trust in its abilities.
- Every contraction brings my baby closer to me.
- I am strong, capable, and ready for this birth.
- I breathe deeply, relaxing my body and mind.
- My body and my baby are working together in harmony.

Active Labor

- Each surge brings me closer to meeting my baby.
- I trust my body's wisdom and let it guide me.
- I surrender to the intensity, knowing it brings my baby closer.
- I breathe through each contraction, releasing tension with every exhale.

- My body is capable of birthing my baby in the most perfect way.

Transition and Pushing

- I am strong and capable, and I trust my body's power.

- My body knows when and how to push my baby out.

- I listen to my body's signals and follow its lead.

- I celebrate each push, knowing I am bringing my baby closer to my arms.

Creating Personalized Affirmations

Now that you've seen examples of affirmations, let's make them personal. Start by identifying what concerns or fears you have about your birth experience. What feels most overwhelming when you think about labor or delivery? Write these fears down—getting them out of your mind and onto paper can be incredibly freeing.

Next, take each fear or worry and reframe it into a positive and empowering statement. For example, if you're worried about not being strong enough, rewrite it as: *"I am strong and capable of birthing my baby."* Or, if you feel uncertain about your body, reframe it as: *"My body was made for this. I trust the process of birth."* These affirmations should resonate with your unique needs, give you confidence, and help shift your mindset toward empowerment.

*My body was made for this,
and I trust its wisdom.*

Affirmation Creation

What is a fear or worry you have about birth?

How can you reframe this fear into a positive and empowering statement?

Note: For example, if your fear is: "I'm worried that I'm not strong enough to get through birth on my own," you can reframe it to: "I am strong and capable of birthing my baby. I trust my body and the tools I have to support me."

Affirmation Creation

What is a fear or worry you have about birth?

How can you reframe this fear into a positive and empowering statement?

Affirmation Creation

What is a fear or worry you have about birth?

How can you reframe this fear into a positive and empowering statement?

Reflection

Which affirmation(s) resonate with you the most? Highlight or circle the one(s) you want to focus on as you prepare for birth.

These affirmations and prompts can help guide you toward a calm, empowered mindset as you prepare for your unique birth journey.

Chapter 31
Crafting Your Birth Plan

BIRTH IS ONE OF the most personal and transformative experiences of your life, and with it comes a variety of options and choices. Many parents are surprised by the sheer number of decisions they may encounter during labor and delivery. Taking the time to explore these options beforehand can help you feel informed, prepared, and empowered as you approach your big day.

To make this process easier, we've organized these options into four categories, each covering a different stage of the birthing experience. Within each category, you'll find a checklist of potential interventions and preferences. Use this as a guide to explore what feels most aligned with your wishes. It's important to remember that no two birth plans will look the same, and that's perfectly okay. Your plan should reflect what feels right for you.

As you work through these checklists, I encourage you to:

- **Research anything you're unsure about.** Use trusted sources, talk to your birth provider, and lean on your support system for insight.

- **Stay true to your preferences.** Birth is personal, and there are no wrong answers.

Parents often find themselves falling into one of three approaches to birth:

1. **Welcoming Interventions:** Open to using available medical tools and technologies.

2. **Go-With-the-Flow:** Flexible and open to decisions as labor progresses.

3. **Minimal Interventions:** Favoring a natural approach with as few interventions as possible.

Whichever approach resonates with you, knowing your options ahead of time will help you feel confident and prepared. When you're ready, use the birth plan summary page to clearly outline your preferences for each stage of labor. This process is not about perfection—it's about ensuring your voice is heard and your values are honored as you bring your baby into the world.

BIRTH PLAN OPTIONS
Checklist

First Stage: Early & Active Labor

Environment & Comfort
- Bathtub or shower access
- Freedom to move, eat, and drink
- Lighting and sound: music, dim lights, quiet, aromatherapy
- Clothing choice: own clothes or hospital gown
- Preference for water breaking naturally

Pain Management Options
- TENS unit
- Nitrous oxide
- Epidural: right away / wait & see / last resort
- Birth comb
- Breathing or visualization techniques
- Warm packs or cool cloths

Partner Support
- Hip compression or counter pressure
- Massage or light touch
- Calm verbal encouragement
- Offering hydration or cool cloths

Medical Preferences
- Fetal monitoring: continuous or intermittent
- Cervical checks: none / limited / as needed
- Pitocin: okay / only if necessary / prefer not
- Water breaking: natural vs. artificial

Movement & Positioning
- Change positions every 20–30 minutes
- Walking, swaying, or standing supported by partner or furniture
- Use of birth ball, peanut ball, or CUB (Comfort Upright Birth) support
- Upright positions such as leaning forward, hands-and-knees, or supported kneeling
- Supported rest positions with pillows or side-lying for recovery between contractions

Notes:

BIRTH PLAN OPTIONS
Checklist

Second Stage: Pushing & Birth

Environment & Comfort
- Bathtub or bed for pushing
- Lighting, music, and room temperature preferences
- Mirror for pushing or visual feedback
- Choice of who is present during birth

Pain Management Options
- Continue chosen method (TENS, Nitrous, Epidural)
- Breathing and visualization guidance
- Warm compresses or perineal support
- Encouragement for rest and focus between contractions

Partner Support
- Verbal coaching and emotional reassurance
- Providing cool cloths or sips of water or ice chips
- Helping with position changes or holding physical support
- Maintaining calm presence and encouragement

Medical Preferences
- Perineal care: massage/stretching or warm compresses
- Vacuum or forceps if needed
- Natural tear vs. episiotomy

Movement & Positioning
- Preferred positions in bed: side-lying, hands-and-knees, upright, reclined, on back
- Option to push in water if available (tub or birth pool)
- Use of birth ball, peanut ball, or CUB (Comfort Upright Birth) support for positioning
- Freedom to push when fully dilated or when the urge is felt
- Adjusting positions for progress and comfort

Notes:

BIRTH PLAN OPTIONS
Checklist

Third Stage: After Birth & Golden Hour

Environment & Bonding
- Immediate skin-to-skin contact (Golden Hour)
- Calm lighting and quiet atmosphere
- Partner or chosen support person present during recovery
- Opportunity for delayed procedures to allow bonding time

Baby Care Options
- Feeding preference: breast or bottle
- Cord clamping: wait 3 minutes or until cord stops pulsing and color drains
- Choice of who cuts the cord
- Placenta: save, encapsulate, or standard disposal
- Baby medications: Vitamin K, Hep B vaccine, and eye ointment — each has a specific purpose; learn what they're for and discuss your preferences with your provider.

Post-Birth Care
- Pitocin for bleeding prevention (routine or by request)
- Gentle perineal care and comfort measures
- In case of emergency, partner to stay with mother or go with baby
- Assessment by a hospital pelvic PT if available

Notes:

A plan is a guide, not a guarantee. Stay flexible, stay focused, and stay empowered.

Chapter 32

What to Pack in Your Hospital (or Birth Center) Bag

Preparing your hospital bag is a practical way to ensure you have everything you need for labor, delivery, and those precious early postpartum moments. This checklist is designed to help you pack thoughtfully, covering both essentials and comfort items. Take the time to review the options, and feel free to personalize the list to match your unique needs and preferences. If you're uncertain about any items, do some research, or consult with your provider to see what might best support you.

Checklist Overview

Here's a summarized list of essential items for labor, delivery, and postpartum:

For Mom

- Comfortable clothes for going home
- Nursing bras, tanks, and breast pads
- Robe, slippers, cozy socks, and pajamas

- Toiletries: toothbrush, lip balm, body wash, etc.
- Snacks, drinks, and a water bottle
- Pillow and blanket from home
- Phone and charger

For Baby

- Going-home outfit (weather-appropriate)
- Receiving blanket and swaddles
- Diapers, wipes, and burp cloths
- Car seat (installed)

Labor Support

- Birth tools/props: TENS unit, rebozo, birth comb, etc.
- Meditative or calming playlists
- Noise-canceling headphones
- Affirmation cards

Documents

- ID, insurance information, and admission form
- Birth plan and pediatrician information

Holistic Items for the Mindful Mom

For those who prefer a holistic approach, consider adding items that promote relaxation, energy, and comfort for both body and mind:

- **Electrolyte Support:** Pack Adrenal Cocktail or an electrolyte powder to maintain hydration and stabilize energy levels.

- **Filtered or Distilled Water:** Bring your preferred water to stay hydrated with added minerals if desired.

- **Essential Oils:** Use cotton balls to apply oils like lavender for relaxation or peppermint for energy. The flexibility of cotton balls makes it easy to adjust scents as needed.

- **Mood Lighting:** Create a calming environment with battery-powered tea light candles, perfect for reducing harsh lighting in the hospital room.

- **High-Protein Snacks:** Stock up on snacks that sustain energy and stabilize blood sugar levels during labor and recovery.

These items are simple yet impactful additions to your hospital bag, helping you feel grounded and supported during this transformative time.

HOSPITAL BAG
Checklist

for mom

- ◯ Robe
- ◯ Swim top (if using tub)
- ◯ Slippers/ Cozy Socks
- ◯ Nursing Bra
- ◯ Nursing Tank
- ◯ Maternity Underwear
- ◯ Nursing Cover
- ◯ Going Home Outfit
- ◯ Jacket
- ◯ Sandals
- ◯ Water Bottle
- ◯ Snacks Loose
- ◯ Pajamas
- ◯ Hair Ties/Clip
- ◯ Hairbrush
- ◯ Lip Balm
- ◯ Nipple Cream
- ◯ Favorite Pillow
- ◯ Makeup
- ◯ Medications
- ◯ Vitamins
- ◯ Phone & Charger

for baby

- ◯ Onesie
- ◯ Mittens
- ◯ Hat/headband
- ◯ Socks
- ◯ Receiving Blanket
- ◯ Swaddle
- ◯ Burp Cloth
- ◯ Pacifier
- ◯ Diapers
- ◯ Baby Wipes
- ◯ Baby Lotion
- ◯ Body Wash/Shampoo
- ◯ Going-Home Outfit
- ◯ Carseat
- ◯ Sound Machine
- ◯ Photo Props

for dad

- ◯ Socks
- ◯ Underwear
- ◯ Sweatpants
- ◯ T-Shirt
- ◯ Sweatshirt
- ◯ Comfortable Shoes
- ◯ Pajamas
- ◯ Snacks & Drinks
- ◯ Phone & Charger
- ◯ Pillow
- ◯ Blanket
- ◯ Towel
- ◯ Jacket
- ◯ Cash

HOSPITAL BAG
Checklist

labor support

- ○ Birth Comb
- ○ Handheld Fan
- ○ Affirmation Cards
- ○ Battery Tea Lights
- ○ Rebozo/Sarong
- ○ Cupping Tool, Balm
- ○ CUB/ Peanut Ball
- ○ TENS unit
- ○ Essential Oils
- ○ Headphones
- ○ Bluetooth Speaker
- ○ Mint Gum

documents

- ○ ID
- ○ Birth Plan
- ○ Pediatrician Info
- ○ Admission Form
- ○ Insurance Information
- ○ Emergency Contacts

toiletries

- ○ Mouthwash
- ○ Toothbrush
- ○ Toothpaste
- ○ Body Wash
- ○ Shampoo
- ○ Conditioner
- ○ Makeup Wipes
- ○ Deodorant
- ○ Moisturizer Body
- ○ Lotion
- ○ Glasses/Contacts
- ○ Face Wash

other

- ○ Book/Kindle
- ○ Ziploc Bags
- ○ Laundry Bag
- ○ Nursing Pillow
- ○ Wallet
- ○ Laptop/Tablet

hospital provides

Diapers	Hat	Perry Bottle
Wipes	Baby Wash	Ice Pack/Pads
Swaddles	Baby Lotion	Birth Ball

Chapter 33

Preparing for Labor:
Foods and Teas to Consider in the Final 4-6 Weeks

The last six weeks of pregnancy are a critical time for preparing the body for labor and delivery. While no specific foods or teas can guarantee an easier labor, some may help support the process by promoting uterine health and providing essential nutrients. Here's a list of foods and teas that are often recommended during the last six weeks of pregnancy to potentially aid in labor preparation:

Foods:

- **Dates:** Consuming dates in the last few weeks of pregnancy is a traditional practice believed to help with cervical dilation and reduce the need for labor induction. Aim for 4-6 dates per day.

- **Protein-Rich Foods:** Foods like lean meats, poultry, fish, eggs, beans, and legumes provide essential amino acids that support muscle strength and stamina during labor.

- **Leafy Greens:** Spinach, kale, and other leafy greens are rich in iron, which can help prevent anemia and maintain energy levels during labor.

- **Whole Grains:** Foods like brown rice, whole wheat pasta, and quinoa provide complex carbohydrates that supply long-lasting energy.

- **Lean Protein and Omega-3s:** Salmon, chia seeds, and flaxseeds are sources of omega-3 fatty acids, which can help reduce inflammation and support overall health.

- **Spices:** Some spices like ginger and turmeric have anti-inflammatory properties and can help alleviate discomfort during labor.

- **Fruits:** Berries, especially strawberries and blueberries, are packed with antioxidants and vitamin C, which promote overall health.

- **Nuts:** Almonds, walnuts, and pistachios provide healthy fats, protein, and energy.

Teas:

- **Red Raspberry Leaf Tea:** This herbal tea is believed to tone the uterine muscles and may help promote more efficient contractions during labor. Start with a small amount and gradually increase intake as your due date approaches.

- **Peppermint Tea:** Peppermint tea can help with digestion and reduce nausea, which can be beneficial during labor.

- **Ginger Tea:** Ginger tea is known for its anti-nausea properties and can be soothing during labor.

- **Nettle Tea:** Nettle tea is a good source of iron, calcium, and magnesium, which can help maintain energy levels and reduce muscle cramps.

- **Chamomile Tea:** Chamomile tea can help with relaxation and stress reduction, which can be useful during the last weeks of pregnancy.

- **Lemon Balm Tea:** Lemon balm is calming and may help with anxiety and stress.

It's important to consult with your healthcare provider or a qualified nutritionist before making significant dietary changes during pregnancy. While these foods and teas are generally considered safe and may provide some benefits, individual responses can vary. Additionally, remember that a healthy and balanced diet throughout pregnancy is essential for overall well-being and the best preparation for labor.

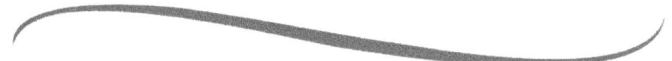

As you move closer to the incredible moment of meeting your baby, take comfort in knowing that the small, intentional steps you take each day can make a world of difference. Whether it's revisiting your birth plan, practicing affirmations, or dedicating a few minutes to your breathing exercises, these mindful moments help prepare both your mind and body for the journey ahead. This consistent focus on your preparation not only nurtures your mental well-being but also builds a sense of calm and confidence as you approach labor.

For all mothers—whether this is your first birth or a chance to create a more empowering experience after a prior one—know that your efforts are creating a strong foundation for a positive, redemptive birth. Picture yourself feeling ready, excited, and supported as you step into this transformative time, knowing you have done everything to prepare for this amazing moment. Trust in your strength, lean into your tools and support, and embrace the beauty of what lies ahead.

Preparation is a mix of practical steps and mental readiness.

Which labor support tools or techniques do you want to practice using before your due date?

What mindset or affirmations will help you stay calm and focused during labor?

Your birth space maters. Reflect on what makes
you feel most at ease and supported.

What details are important to you for your birth?

Preparation is a mix of practical steps and mental readiness.

Which labor support tools or techniques do you want to practice using before your due date?

What mindset or affirmations will help you stay calm and focused during labor?

SECTION IV: Postpartum Recovery

Welcoming a new baby into your life is an extraordinary experience, but it also comes with significant changes for your body, mind, and emotions. While preparing for your baby is exciting, it's equally important to prioritize your own recovery and well-being during the postpartum period. This section is dedicated to guiding you through the essentials of postpartum recovery, from the first few weeks to the months that follow. You'll find practical advice, recipes, journal prompts, and supportive strategies to help you heal, rebuild your strength, and navigate this transformative time with confidence and care. Remember, taking care of yourself is not a luxury—it's essential for thriving in your new role as a mother.

Essentials for the Initial 2-3 Weeks

Having a baby is quite the life experience. While it is exciting to prepare for our babies and shop for their nursery and pick out cute baby clothes, it is *imperative* that we *also* prepare to care for ourselves! This list covers most everything that you may need.

Postpartum Care At-Home Checklist

Clothing

- Robe
- Nursing Tanks (3)
- Nursing Bras (1-sleep, 2-day)
- Nursing PJs (1-2)
- Maternity/ Postpartum Underwear
- Nursing Cover (if guests visiting)
- Nursing friendly tops
- Elastic Waist Loose/Comfy Bottoms

Nipple Care

- Nipple cream or coconut oil (**Bonus:** A couple drops of Geranium and Roman Camomile essential oils can be added to the coconut oil for healing and pain)
- Nipple pads (organic cotton)
- Silverettes (to help chafed nipples heal between feedings)

Postpartum Care At-Home Checklist

Down There & Belly Care

- ○ Perineal Ice Packs
- ○ Witch Hazel Pads
- ○ Dermoplast or Earth Mama Perineal Spray
- ○ Frida Mom Peri Bottle
- ○ Epsom Salts or Herbal Bath Mix
- ○ Pads: Look for organic pads without top weaving that may catch on stitches if present
- ○ Optional: Organic disposable postpartum underwear
- ○ Basic Abdominal Binder: only for first few weeks, discontinue use if it causes downward pressure on pelvic floor

Nutrition/ Hydration

- ○ Filtered Water
- ○ Adrenal Cocktail/ Electrolytes
- ○ Favorite LARGE water bottle
- ○ Prepare protein-rich snacks for nursing to stabilize blood sugar and support healing. Check the recipe section for high-protein no-bake lactation bites—perfect to make ahead and freeze before your due date.
- ○ Prepare at least a week's worth of protein-rich meals to freeze before your due date. Consider setting up a meal train, as cooking nutritious meals during the first 2–3 weeks postpartum can be incredibly challenging.

Rest isn't just recovery—it's rebuilding. I give myself the grace to heal.

Chapter 34
5-5-5 Rule

EMBRACING A GENTLE JOURNEY into motherhood is essential, and the 5-5-5 Postpartum Recovery Rule offers a nurturing pathway to bond with your newborn while safeguarding your health. This thoughtful approach supports your healing, helps prevent postpartum complications like depression, anxiety, and mastitis, and strengthens your connections with your baby and family.

5 Days in Bed

Your first five days at home are for deep rest and bonding. This time is about you and your baby together, lying in bed, engaging in plenty of skin-to-skin contact, and establishing breastfeeding. Allow yourself to nap, read, and soak in these precious moments. It's a time to be cared for as much as you care for your new baby, so let your partner or another support person cater to your needs by bringing meals and water directly to you. Surrender to being pampered—it's not only allowed, it's recommended!

5 Days on the Bed

As you transition to the next phase, you'll still be on the bed but might start sitting up and engaging in light activities. Continue those invaluable cuddle sessions with your baby, which not only strengthen your bond but also enhance oxytocin release, aiding both emotional connection and breastfeeding. If you have another child, this is a wonderful opportunity to connect with them too, perhaps by reading stories together, working on puzzles, or drawing. It's important to remain mindful of your recovery and not overextend yourself during these activities.

5 Days Around the Bed

Now you can gently increase your mobility by standing and moving around the bed. Feel free to engage in very light tasks like folding laundry, always listening to your body's signals. Limit standing to short periods, ideally no more than 30 minutes at a time, to avoid strain. Your primary focus should still be on recovery and rest.

The 5-5-5 Rule is a loving framework that respects the profound changes your body and spirit undergo after birth. Integrating this rule into your recovery plan not only prioritizes your well-being but also enhances the well-being of your entire family. Remember, allowing yourself this time to heal and bond is one of the most loving actions you can take as a new mother.

Slow and steady wins the postpartum race. I honor my body's pace.

Chapter 35

Supporting Your Recovery: Signs to Watch, Self-Care, and When to Seek Medical Care

Excessive bleeding after 1 week

NORMAL POSTPARTUM BLOOD LOSS, also known as lochia, occurs after giving birth and typically consists of three stages:

1. **Lochia Rubra:** This is the first stage, which occurs during the first 3 to 5 days after childbirth. It consists of bright red blood and may contain small clots. The amount of blood loss during this stage can vary, but it's generally considered normal as long as it's not excessive.

2. **Lochia Serosa:** This stage follows the rubra stage and typically lasts from about day 4 to day 10 postpartum. The color of the discharge changes to pink or brownish, and it may also contain some mucus. The volume of blood decreases during this stage.

3. **Lochia Alba:** This is the final stage, lasting from around day 10 to 6 weeks postpartum. The discharge becomes lighter in color, resembling white or yellowish discharge. It may appear similar to the discharge at the end of a menstrual period.

The amount of normal postpartum blood loss can vary from woman to woman, but a general guideline is that any bleeding that doesn't exceed the flow of a heavy menstrual period is considered normal. In the first few days after childbirth, bleeding may be heavier, but it should gradually decrease as the weeks go by.

It's important to note that while some bleeding is normal, excessive bleeding can be a sign of a postpartum hemorrhage, which is a potentially serious medical condition. Signs of excessive bleeding and potential postpartum hemorrhage include:

- Soaking through a menstrual pad in an hour or less.

- Passing large blood clots, especially if they are bigger than a golf ball.

- Feeling lightheaded, dizzy, or faint.

- Rapid heart rate.

- Pale or clammy skin.

- A sudden gush of bright red bleeding.

If you experience any of these symptoms, it's important to seek immediate medical attention. Postpartum hemorrhage can be caused by various factors, including uterine atony (failure of the uterus to contract after delivery), retained placental fragments, tears in the birth canal, or certain medical conditions.

Always consult with your healthcare provider if you have concerns about your postpartum bleeding or if you're unsure whether the amount of blood loss you're experiencing is normal. They can provide you with personalized guidance based on your individual circumstances.

Fever of 100 or greater

In the early postpartum stage, which refers to the period shortly after childbirth, it's common for a woman's body temperature to fluctuate. Hormonal changes, including the process of the body expelling excess fluids, can influence body temperature.

A normal body temperature for a postpartum woman is generally considered to be in the range of 97°F to 99°F (36.1°C to 37.2°C). A fever is generally defined as a body temperature of 100.4°F (38°C) or higher. In the postpartum period, a fever can be a sign of infection, which is a concern because the body's immune system is more vulnerable during this time due to the recent delivery and potential changes in immune function.

It's always best to reach out to a healthcare professional if you have concerns about your body temperature or any other symptoms you're experiencing in the postpartum period. They can provide you with appropriate guidance based on your specific situation.

Severe Headache

If you experience a severe headache in the early postpartum period, especially if it's accompanied by other symptoms such as visual disturbances, high blood pressure, nausea, vomiting, confusion, seizures, or any other concerning symptoms, it's important to seek medical attention promptly. Your healthcare provider can evaluate your symptoms, perform necessary tests, and determine the appropriate course of action.

Constipation and Hemorrhoids

Constipation and hemorrhoids are common issues that can occur in the postpartum period. While they may be uncomfortable and inconvenient, they should not be ignored due to potential complications and the impact they can have on a person's overall well-being. Here's a brief explanation of why they should not be ignored and what can be done for treatment:

Constipation

Constipation can be exacerbated by factors like hormonal changes, dehydration, pain from childbirth, and certain medications taken during the postpartum period. Ignoring constipation can lead to increased discomfort, straining during bowel movements (which can be painful if you've had perineal tears or an episiotomy), and even the development of hemorrhoids.

Hemorrhoids

Hemorrhoids are swollen blood vessels in the rectal area that can result from straining during bowel movements, increased pressure on the rectal veins during pregnancy, and childbirth itself. Ignoring hemorrhoids can lead to increased pain, bleeding, itching, and potential complications like thrombosis (blood clot formation) within the hemorrhoid.

Home Treatment for Constipation and Hemorrhoids:

- **Hydration:** Drinking plenty of water with electrolytes to help soften stools and prevent constipation.

- **Magnesium glycinate:** known for helping with stress and muscle tension.

- **Magnesium Citrate:** known for adding water to the stool. Dosage is typically recommended to be titrated based on the amount needed to result in a healthy bowel movement. People usually take the smallest dose and wait 24 hours. Dosage is increased each day until stool is healthy like a soft banana. Only take magnesium citrate as needed and not as a daily supplement.

- **Incorporating Daily Movement and Belly Breathing Throughout Your Day:** Both are key for improving digestion and gut motility.

- **Fiber-Rich Diet**: Consuming foods high in fiber, such as whole grains, fruits, vegetables, and legumes, can help promote regular bowel movements.

- **Kiwi Fruit**: Kiwi fruit has recently gained attention as an effective natural remedy for managing constipation, often outperforming traditional treatments like MiraLAX and psyllium. Research indicates that consuming two kiwis daily can significantly improve bowel movements and reduce symptoms of constipation. This is due to the high fiber content and unique enzymes in kiwi, which promote regularity without the bloating or discomfort sometimes associated with other laxatives. Studies have shown that kiwi not only improves stool consistency but also enhances patient satisfaction, making it a preferred choice for those seeking a natural and gentle solution to constipation.

- **Stool Softeners**: Over-the-counter stool softeners can help alleviate constipation and reduce straining.

- **Topical Treatment**: Over-the-counter hemorrhoid creams or ointments can help alleviate itching and discomfort.

- **Essential oils:** Are known to relieve discomfort, reduce inflammation and pain. Essential oils including tea tree (clinically proven effective for hemorrhoids), lavender (calming), Frankincense (anti-inflammatory, anti-fungal, anti-bacterial) can be a powerful combination to help resolve hemorrhoid discomfort and help with healing. They can be combined in a roller ball with fractionated coconut oil and applied to fingers and then applied to affected tissue. Can also put these oils into a dropper bottle and saturate onto a cloth and "tuck" it over the tissue till the blend has absorbed. Be sure to use only oils that are third party tested for purity and used in university research such as doTerra. The following would be one example of how one would dilute these in a 10 ml roller ball: 5 drops each of tea tree, Frankincense and Lavender. Fill the rest of the roller ball with organic fractionated coconut oil.

- **Sitz Baths**: Soaking in warm water can soothe hemorrhoids and provide relief. You could put a few drops of the above essential oils into a container with a teaspoon of coconut oil before adding to the sitz bath.

- **Note**: Our best time to have a bowel movement is within 30 minutes of our first meal of the day. Typically drinking a warm drink in the morning and then sitting on the toilet using a squatty potty or stool under feet. Take 5 minutes to belly breathe, allowing the belly to expand/relax with inhales slowly. This is a great lifelong habit.

When to Seek Professional Help: *If constipation or hemorrhoids persist despite home remedies, or if you experience severe pain, bleeding, or any unusual symptoms, it's important to consult a healthcare provider.*

Incontinence after week 3

It's important not to dismiss persistent urinary incontinence after 3 weeks postpartum, as it could have implications for your overall health and quality of life.

A pelvic floor physical therapist or pelvic floor occupational therapist is your first line of care with any issues with bladder or bowel control issues. They can provide a thorough assessment and customize the appropriate treatment plan based on their objective findings. As there are many reasons for us to experience loss of bladder or bowel control, there are many different treatment options. It is crucial that women are not told to just "do Kegels" by repetitively contracting their pelvic floor when the cause of leakage can actually be excessive pelvic floor muscle tension.

Note: In the postpartum period, I find that some women's pelvic floor muscles will go into a "freeze" pattern where they will feel disconnected and weak ***or*** their muscles will go into "fight" patterning where the muscles get stuck in a state of tension. Both patterns can result in bladder leakage, so it becomes essential to be evaluated by a pelvic health expert that can determine what your pattern is to be able to resolve the symptoms effectively.

Painful Sex *(wait the 6 weeks or more)*

After childbirth, up to 50% of women may experience pain during sexual intercourse, a condition known as dyspareunia. This can be due to a combination of physical and psychological factors related to pregnancy, delivery, and postpartum changes.

Common reasons for postpartum pain during sex include:

Trauma to the Pelvic Area: Vaginal delivery, especially if there were tears, episiotomies, or the need for forceps or vacuum assistance, can cause physical trauma to the pelvic floor muscles and tissues.

- **Hormonal Changes**: Hormonal fluctuations during and after pregnancy can lead to vaginal dryness and decreased lubrication, making intercourse uncomfortable or painful.

- **Scar Tissue Formation**: Healing from perineal tears or episiotomies can result in scar tissue formation, which can cause tightness and discomfort during penetration.

- **Muscle Tension and Spasm**: The pelvic floor muscles may become tense or spasmodic due to the stress of childbirth or holding tension during the healing process. This can also occur after cesarean section births due to the muscle and fascial connections of the deep core system.

- **Psychological Factors**: Anxiety, fear, and apprehension related to the postpartum body, pain, or changes in sexual function can contribute to pain during sex.

Pelvic therapists can help women find the underlying issues leading to their pain with sex and help make a plan to resolve it. It is ideal to not expect to be sexually active for the first 6 weeks postpartum at a minimum during the time that our muscles and tissues are still healing after childbirth. Many women wait to see their pelvic therapist to have a pelvic floor assessment before planning to have sex again. In this visit, pelvic therapists can also go over strategies to reduce any pelvic pain with vaginal penetration in the early postpartum period.

Pelvic heaviness/pressure

A newly postpartum woman should not ignore symptoms of pelvic pressure or heaviness because these symptoms can indicate underlying issues that require attention such as pelvic organ prolapse or pelvic floor dysfunction. Addressing symptoms early can help prevent potential complications down the line. Pelvic floor issues, if left untreated, can lead to more serious problems over time.

Remember that postpartum recovery is a unique experience for each woman, and seeking assistance for any discomfort or symptoms you're experiencing is crucial for your well-being. If you're feeling pelvic pressure or heaviness after childbirth, consulting with your healthcare provider or a pelvic therapist can help you determine the cause and develop a plan to address and manage these symptoms effectively.

Chapter 36
Postpartum Recovery in Weeks 0-6
The Core Four

THESE FOUR CATEGORIES ENCOMPASS essential aspects of the early postpartum period. Prioritizing proper nutrition, core engagement, physical support, and pelvic floor care can contribute to a smoother recovery process and help you regain strength and comfort after childbirth.

1. Nutrition/Hydration:

Proper nutrition and hydration are essential for postpartum recovery. Adequate nutrients and fluids support healing, energy levels, and breastfeeding if applicable. Focus on a balanced diet rich in fruits, vegetables, clean proteins, whole grains, and healthy fats. Staying hydrated is crucial for overall well-being and helps with milk production if breastfeeding.

2. Core Breathing:

Core breathing involves engaging the deep core muscles, including the diaphragm, transverse abdominis, and pelvic floor muscles. Practicing gentle and coordinated breathing techniques can help restore proper core function, stabilize the pelvis, and support healing. This can aid in preventing or addressing issues like diastasis recti (abdominal separation) and pelvic floor dysfunction.

Core breathing means mindfully allowing your ribs, abdominals and pelvic floor to release and lengthen with your *inhale,* and slowly engaging them to draw up and in with *exhale.* Think of the extremes of breath (inhale/expand vs exhale/recoil or shorten) like working to regain the ability to fully bend and straighten your elbow before picking up a heavy weight to do biceps curls. You can work on this while nursing or holding your baby in sitting, while laying on your side, standing leaning over your kitchen counter, or on your hands and knees.

Changing the position you have your body in will change the area that gets expanding with inhale and demand on your core muscles. Reclined will be easiest and on your hands and knees will be more challenging. Doing a couple sets of 5 core breaths in different postures throughout the day to check in and connect with your core is the goal. This is **not** the time to start a core exercise video or app program geared towards the general population. Rest wins the day at this point in your recovery!

In early postpartum, the area of our body that will need the most breath attention to help release and *expand* will be the lower posterior rib cage and low back.

A breathing position to try: sit on a cushion criss cross, lean your left forearm on your left knee and place your right hand on your right lower ribs. Take slow 4 count inhales focused on expanding the ribs under your right hand. Repeat on both sides. Another option is while in a car, take a few breaths while trying to press your low back into the lumbar support as you work to create length and expand your posterior lower ribs.

3. Decompression:

In the weeks following childbirth, it's essential to prioritize the healing process for your pelvic floor, abdominal wall, and pelvic organs. To relieve pressure in the pelvic area and spine, consider gentle decompression techniques. These techniques include lying down with hips raised on one or two pillows and propping your legs on a couch or up against a wall, which can promote circulation and reduce swelling, discomfort, and stress.

For c-section recovery, it is also essential to not be upright for too long without horizontal breaks as it will create excessive pulling on the healing skin and fascia just above the incision and can lead to an undesirable bulge above the scar later on.

It's important to note that caring for a newborn will require a lot of forward posture time, leading to neck, upper back, and pelvic floor strain. To help your body recover and minimize the strain, try to get into a decompression posture twice a day for 5-10 minutes. This can be as simple as lying flat on your back with no pillows under your head and legs propped up on pillows or a couch, or you can elevate your hips with a couple of pillows under your hips and legs up against the wall. Let your partner know that this is a self care goal and that you may need their support with baby care for you to be able to make this goal a reality.

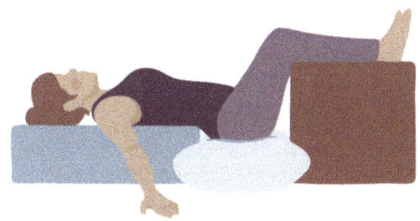

4. Pelvic Floor Safety:

Paying attention to your pelvic floor health is crucial during early postpartum recovery. Avoid activities that place any strain on the pelvic floor, such as being on your feet for prolonged periods (in the first 3 weeks, you really shouldn't be going for outdoor walks yet), heavy lifting, intense abdominal exercises, and high-impact activities. Your internal ligaments that support your organs are in a phase of healing and returning to a non stretched out state. It's crucial that you know that no amount of positive mindset, focus on how strong your were before birth, etc. will change the fact that your ligaments need t to heal. Gradually reintroduce physical activity, focusing on pelvic floor-safe exercises like gentle walking after 3 weeks, kegel exercises, and guided pelvic floor strengthening.

Note: Your family members may need to be made aware of the fact that your internal ligaments are not able to support your organs fully in the first month. Even if you are looking great on the outside, your body still needs time.

In general, you should not feel a downward pressure or strain in your pelvic floor with *any* activities. If you do experience this, you should work to modify the activity or avoid it until you have worked with a pelvic floor specialist. A good rule of thumb to help support your pelvic floor and core with activity is to "Exhale with Effort" and avoid holding your breath with activity.

A pelvic floor therapist can be your greatest support in safely and positively regaining your previous activities and more. Working with a pelvic therapist is beneficial when aiming to resume activities like lifting and running. Investing time with these specialists will bring long-term benefits.

Hydration, nutrition, movement, and rest—the pillars of my healing.

Chapter 37

Postpartum Nutrition

For a new mother, it is normal to feel overwhelmed with caring for your baby in addition to caring for yourself. Here's a summary of the best foods to focus on in the early postpartum period:

Balanced Meals: Aim for balanced meals with clean, high-quality proteins like grass-fed organic beef and organic chicken, whole grains (brown rice, oats), and lots of colorful fruits and veggies.

Protein:

Conventional sources recommend that postpartum and breastfeeding women need between 50-75 grams of protein a day. I would recommend aiming for at least 75 grams, and even aiming for 90-100 grams/day. On pages 229-230, there's a breakdown of protein content in various sources. Keep this table in mind when working to get adequate protein on a daily basis which will be crucial to help your tissues heal, reduce inflammation, help your hormone balance, reduce sugar and carb cravings, and balance your blood sugar.

Healthy Fats: Include good fats like avocados, nuts, and olive oil for energy and well-being.

Hydration: Shoot for drinking at least half your bodyweight in ounces of water per day and add in electrolytes daily. Adrenal cocktail by Jigsaw has the perfect combination of sodium and potassium and has the addition of whole food vitamin C that in combination supports your adrenals in this time of stress on the body as you recover from childbirth and manage the care of your newborn. You can take adrenal cocktail 2-3 times a day to support your electrolyte needs.

Easy Snacks: Nuts, pumpkin seeds, yogurt, and fruit make simple and nutritious snacks. The bonus with pumpkin seeds is that they are a great source of magnesium which is crucial in this phase.

Iron and Omega-3s: Eat iron-rich foods like lean meats and add omega-3 sources like fatty fish or seeds.

Simple Options: Opt for easy-to-digest foods like soups, smoothies, and well-cooked veggies.

Gentle on Tummy: Choose foods that are kind to your stomach as you recover. In traditional Ayurvedic medicine, cooked vegetables and fruits are easier to digest than raw.

Listen to Yourself: Pay attention to your body's signals and eat what feels nourishing.

Try to Limit Sugar: Unfortunately, excess sugar can really add fuel to the hormone fire. Keeping blood sugar levels from spiking will best support reducing inflammation and hormonal re-balancing. I really like these two tips for carbs.

> 1. Never have a "naked carb." Meaning don't consume carbs alone. Eat them *with* a good quantity of protein to help maintain balanced blood sugar.

2. Go for a short walk (when able postpartum) after your highest carb meal.

Remember, this time is about taking care of yourself and your little one. Small, nutritious choices can go a long way in supporting your recovery and well-being.

High Protein Food Chart
Animal and Vegan Options

Protein is essential during pregnancy, helping your body build your baby's tissues, repair your own, balance hormones, and keep your energy steady. Most women need a minimum of 75 grams daily—and often more—but many aren't keeping track of how much they're actually getting. It's common to think you've had "some protein" with a meal when the total may fall short. Use this guide to help you track and choose protein-rich foods so you can feel confident you're getting what your body and baby truly need each day.

Food Source	Grams of Protein
3.5 ounces of chicken breast	30 grams protein
3 ounces of beef sirloin	26 grams protein
Equip Foods Protein Powder (1 serving)	21 grams protein
¾ cup Greek Yogurt	17-18 grams protein
½ cup low fat cottage cheese	14 grams protein
1 cup milk	8 grams protein
1 egg	6-7 grams protein

High Protein Food Chart
Animal and Vegan Options

Food Source	Grams of Protein
100 grams broccoli	2.5 grams protein
2 TBS almond butter	7 grams protein
½ avocado	2 grams protein
½ cup lentils	9 grams protein
½ cup soybeans	15 grams protein
100 grams chickpeas	15 grams protein
¼ cup Quinoa	6 grams protein
3oz tempeh	18 grams protein
1 cup cooked black beans	15 grams protein
3 TBS hemp seeds	9.5 grams protein
½ cup tofu	22 grams protein

Chapter 38
Favorite Postpartum Recipes

H**ERE ARE 11 SIMPLE** and nutritious snack and meal recipes for postpartum women in the first 6 weeks after childbirth. These recipes are designed to provide sufficient protein to support healthy blood sugar balance and curb carbohydrate and sugar cravings. I've included a no-bake lactation bite recipe as well:

Protein-Packed Overnight Oats

Ingredients:

- 1/2 cup rolled oats
- 1 cup Greek yogurt
- 2 tablespoons almond butter
- 1 tablespoon chia seeds
- 1 teaspoon honey

Chocolate Protein Greek Yogurt

Ingredients:

- 3/4 cup plain Greek yogurt (18+ grams protein)

- 1 scoop chocolate protein powder (18-20 grams protein)
- Sliced strawberries, bananas or granola for topping

Mix Greek yogurt and protein powder until well combined. Top with sliced fruit.

Egg Burrito

Ingredients:

- 2-3 large eggs
- 1 whole-grain tortilla
- 1/4 cup black beans, drained and rinsed
- Salsa (optional)
- Sliced avocado (optional)
- Shredded cheese (optional)

Scramble the eggs and cook until they are set. Warm the tortilla and place the scrambled eggs, black beans, salsa, avocado, and cheese (if desired) in the center. Roll it up into a burrito and enjoy.

Avocado and Cottage Cheese Toast

Ingredients:

- 1 whole wheat toast

- 1/2 avocado, mashed

- 1/2 cup low-fat cottage cheese

- Sprinkle of black pepper and salt

No-Bake Lactation Bites

Ingredients:

- 1 cup rolled oats

- 1/2 cup almond butter

- 1/4 cup honey

- 1/4 cup ground flaxseed

- 1/4 cup brewer's yeast (lactation aid)

- 1/2 cup chocolate chips (optional)

Mix all ingredients until combined. Roll into 1½-inch balls. Freeze for 10 minutes, then store in the refrigerator. Enjoy cold.

Turkey and Veggie Wrap

Ingredients:

- 1 whole-grain wrap

- 3 slices of turkey breast

- Sliced cucumber, bell peppers, and spinach

- Hummus for spread

Protein-Packed Smoothie

Ingredients:

- 1 cup spinach
- 1/2 banana
- 1/2 cup Greek yogurt
- 1 scoop of protein powder (choose a postpartum-friendly brand)
- 1 tablespoon almond butter
- 1/2 cup almond milk

Egg Salad Sandwich

Ingredients:

- 2 boiled eggs, chopped
- 2 tablespoons Greek yogurt
- Chopped celery and red onion
- Salt and pepper to taste
- Whole-grain bread

Mix eggs, Greek yogurt, celery, and red onion; season to taste and serve on whole-grain bread.

Tuna and White Bean Salad

Ingredients:

- 1 can of tuna, drained
- 1 can of white beans, drained and rinsed
- Chopped cucumber, cherry tomatoes, and red onion
- Olive oil and lemon juice dressing

Combine all ingredients in a bowl. Toss gently with olive oil and lemon juice to taste. Serve immediately or chilled.

Cottage Cheese and Fruit Bowl

Ingredients:

- 1 cup low-fat cottage cheese
- Sliced peaches, pineapple, and kiwi
- Sprinkle of cinnamon

Baked Sweet Potato Fries

Ingredients:

- 2 sweet potatoes, cut into fries
- 1 tablespoon olive oil

- Salt, pepper, and paprika to taste

These recipes provide a variety of options for postpartum women to maintain their energy levels, satisfy cravings, and support lactation. Remember to consult with a healthcare professional for personalized dietary guidance during the postpartum period.

Chapter 39
Lactation Support

Breastfeeding Recommendations from the World Health Organization (WHO)

THE WHO PROVIDES EVIDENCE-BASED guidelines for breastfeeding to promote the health and well-being of both mothers and infants. These recommendations include:

- **Exclusive Breastfeeding:** The WHO recommends exclusive breastfeeding for the first six months of a baby's life. This means that infants receive only breast milk, with no other foods or liquids (including water) except for prescribed medicines and vitamin or mineral supplements.

- **Continued Breastfeeding:** After the first six months, the WHO advises that breastfeeding should continue alongside the introduction of complementary foods for up to two years or more. Breast milk remains an essential source of nutrition and immune protection.

- **On-Demand Feeding:** Infants should be breastfed on demand, as often as they want, day and night. This helps establish and maintain milk production and ensures that the baby receives enough nourishment.

- **Proper Latching:** Ensuring a proper latch is crucial for successful breastfeeding. The baby's mouth should cover as much of the areola (the darker area around the nipple) as possible, not just the nipple itself. A good latch helps prevent nipple pain and ensures the baby gets enough milk.

- **Skin-to-Skin Contact:** Immediate skin-to-skin contact between the mother and newborn is encouraged after birth. This promotes bonding and helps initiate breastfeeding. Babies placed skin-to-skin are more likely to latch on and breastfeed successfully in the first hour of life.

General Guidance for Successful Breastfeeding:

- **Seek Professional Support:** If needed, consult with a lactation consultant or healthcare provider to address any breastfeeding challenges, such as latching difficulties or low milk supply. Early intervention can help resolve issues and promote breastfeeding success.

- **Feed on Demand:** Respond promptly to your baby's hunger cues, which may include rooting, sucking motions, or restlessness. Feeding on demand helps establish and maintain a good milk supply.

- **Positioning:** Find a comfortable breastfeeding position that works for both you and your baby. Common positions include cradle hold, football hold, and side-lying. Experiment to see which one feels most natural.

- **Nutrition and Hydration:** Maintain a balanced diet, stay well-hydrated, and get plenty of rest to support your own health and milk production. It's important for breastfeeding mothers to eat nutritious foods and drink fluids regularly.

- **Bonding and Skin-to-Skin:** Spend time bonding with your baby through skin-to-skin contact, cuddling, and eye contact. These activities can strengthen the emotional connection between you and your infant.

- **Pump and Store Milk:** If you need to be away from your baby, consider pumping and storing breast milk in a clean container. Follow proper storage guidelines to ensure the milk remains safe for your baby.

- **Be Patient:** Breastfeeding can be challenging at times, especially in the early weeks. Be patient with yourself and your baby. It's okay to seek help and take breaks when needed.

Remember that every breastfeeding journey is unique, and it's essential to make choices that work best for you and your baby. A list of resources on lactation are listed at the end of this book.

Chapter 40
Early Core Restoration

Start with Breathing:

Breathing is the foundation of core rehabilitation in the early postpartum phase. After childbirth, especially if you've had a cesarean section or significant abdominal separation (diastasis recti), the abdominal muscles and the pelvic floor muscles can be weakened or compromised. Proper breathing techniques can help activate and engage these muscles while protecting the healing process.

Begin with diaphragmatic breathing, which involves inhaling deeply through your nose, allowing your diaphragm to lower, and expanding your ribcage and lower abdomen. As you exhale, gently engage your pelvic floor and transverse abdominis (deep core muscle) to support your abdominal area. This breathing technique helps re-establish the connection between your core muscles and pelvic floor.

Find Your Alignment:

Posture and alignment play a crucial role in early postpartum recovery. Pay attention to your posture when breastfeeding, holding your baby, and during everyday activities. Engage your core gently to support your spine and pelvis.

By the end of pregnancy, our bodies have adjusted our alignment quite a bit to accommodate our growing baby which will include a flared rib cage in front, and an extended and shortened spine and back muscles. Along with this alignment change comes weakened abdominals and glutes and short and tight low back muscles.

My two favorite ways to help new moms find a more neutral alignment again are:

1. Laying flat on your back with legs elevated (remember the decompression posture from before?) for 5 minutes at a time to allow gravity to elongate the spine.

2. Lean your back up against a wall with feet about 18" away and knees softly bent. Working to touch the back of your head down to your tailbone to the wall while taking 4 slow belly breaths.

I have cared for numerous women over the years who, even 10, 20, or 30 years after childbirth, have not regained their pre-pregnancy body alignment. This has led to years of back tension and a sense that their abdominal muscles may never fully recover.

Think about seeking advice from a pelvic physical therapist who can evaluate your alignment and offer suggestions on how to enhance it. They can also assess any pelvic floor issues, such as weakness or heightened muscle tension, and offer specific exercises or techniques to target these concerns.

Taking Short Strolls:

In the early postpartum phase (after 3 weeks), light physical activity like walking can be beneficial. Start with short, leisurely walks and gradually increase the duration and distance as your body permits. Walking promotes circulation, aids in healing, and can be a gentle way to rebuild stamina.

Focus on maintaining good posture and engaging your core muscles during walks. It's important to listen to your body and rest when needed, especially in the first few weeks postpartum. If you feel any heaviness in your pelvic floor region, this is your body letting you know that it is time to get horizontal for 10-15 minutes to let your pelvic ligaments reset and rest.

Don't Be Afraid to Do Gentle, Non-Loaded Exercises Before 6 Weeks:

While it's essential to respect the initial healing period, gentle, non-loaded exercises can be introduced before the six-week mark. These exercises, such as gentle stretches, deep breathing, and isometric contractions (tightening a muscle without moving the body), can help maintain muscle tone and improve circulation without straining the healing tissues.

But in all honesty, caring for your baby (or babies) is a *lot* of physical work! When lifting and lowering your baby, I highly recommend **exhaling with effort** to help support your core and pelvic floor.

Always consult with your healthcare provider or a pelvic physical/occupational therapist before starting any exercise program, especially in the early postpartum phase. They can provide personalized guidance based on your specific recovery needs and any potential complications from childbirth.

Early postpartum core recovery should prioritize proper breathing, alignment, and gradual progression of exercises while listening to your body's cues. Seek professional guidance to ensure a safe and effective recovery process tailored to your unique needs.

More Strenuous Exercises After 6 Weeks with Core/Hip Foundation Focus:

Around six weeks postpartum, most women receive clearance from their healthcare provider to gradually resume more strenuous exercises. However, it's essential to prioritize rebuilding your core and hip foundation before diving into higher-intensity activities.

Begin with gentle core-strengthening exercises that target the deep abdominals and pelvic floor muscles. Hands and knees belly breathing (lifting your belly with exhale and dropping belly with inhale), pelvic tilts (exhale while flattening low back to floor), and pelvic floor activation with breathing can be beneficial. Incorporate hip-strengthening exercises like mini squats and small staggered lunges to support your core stability. Balancing on one leg and engaging your glutes on the supporting leg while brushing your teeth is a fantastic way to incorporate strength training into a hectic day with a baby.

A great way to improve your posture during walks is by thinking "tall" while setting your rib cage slightly downward to reduce the distance between your ribs and pelvis bones at the front. This technique will engage your core muscles without the need to "suck it in."

Remember that progression should be gradual and guided by your body's readiness. Consult with your pelvic physical therapist with expertise in postpartum recovery to ensure you're doing exercises safely and effectively.

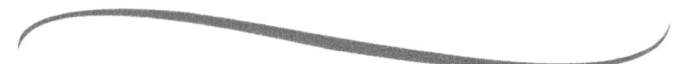

New Mom Stretch Guide

By around three months postpartum, many moms begin to notice ongoing tension in the neck, shoulders, and upper back. Feeding, holding, rocking, and carrying a baby place repeated demands on these areas, often without much recovery time.

On the following pages, you'll find **7 simple stretches** many moms find helpful for easing this tension. I recommend trying all of them first, then returning to the ones that feel the most relieving for your body. You don't need to do them all every time—use this guide as a supportive tool you can come back to as needed.

New Mom Stretches

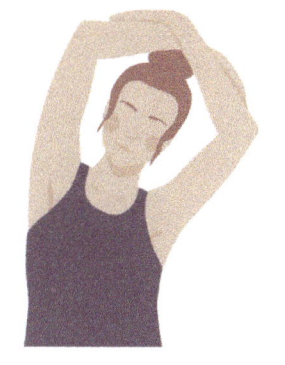

Overhead Side Bend
With arms folded overhead, gently bend to the right, holding for a breath, then repeat to the left. Keep your ribs down and avoid arching your back. 1-3 times on each side.

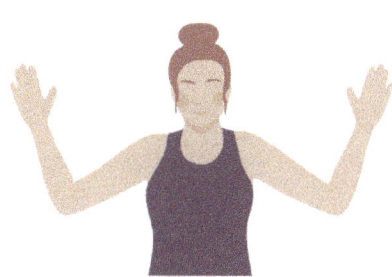

W Stretch
With arms in shape of a "W" palms forward sitting tall, move hands and shoulders back to feel a stretch in front of shoulders & chest without arching your spine. Hold for 2-3 slow breaths.

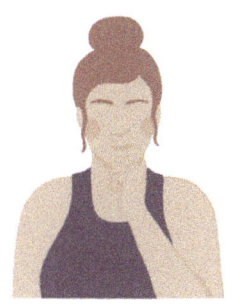

Chin Tuck
Sitting tall, bring your chin back and down slightly to feel a stretch in the base of your neck. Hold 5 seconds, repeat 5 times.

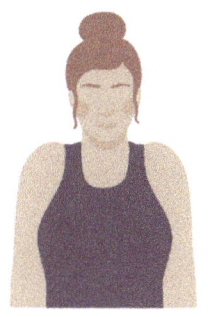

Shoulder Circles
Sit tall with your hands relaxed on your lap. Gently lift your shoulders up toward your ears, roll them back, and lower them down. Repeat this backward circle 5 times.

New Mom Stretches

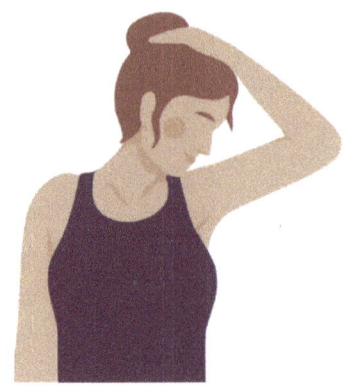

Overhead Side Bend
With arms folded overhead, gently bend to the right, holding for a breath, then repeat to the left. Keep your ribs down and avoid arching your back. 1-3 times on each side.

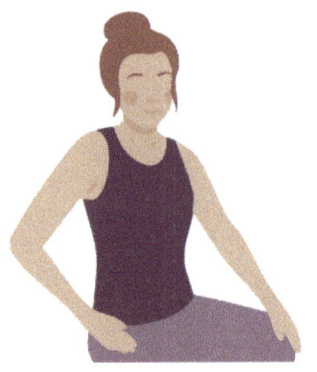

Seated Spine Twist
Sitting tall with hands on your lap, slide one hand forward and the other back to gently twist through your spine. Keep your shoulders relaxed and hold each side for a slow inhale and exhale. Repeat 3–4 times on each side.

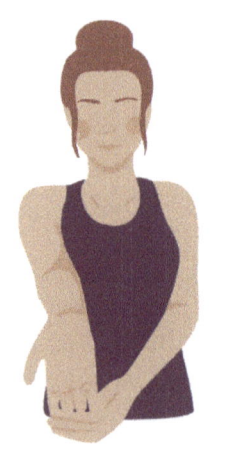

Forearm Stretch
Extend one arm in front of you and gently pull back your fingertips to stretch the front of your forearm. Stay for a breath and repeat both sides.

Rebuilding is a journey, not a sprint. Start small and trust the process.

Chapter 41

When to See a Pelvic Physical or Occupational Therapist Postpartum

IF YOU ARE READING this *after* your birth—congratulations! You did it. If you're still preparing for birth, I am rooting for you and your positive experience. But no matter where you are in your journey, I want you to know this: your early postpartum care is just as important as all the work you are doing now.

If you've had a baby before, you already know how those first few weeks can feel. The focus is almost entirely on your newborn—doctor's visits to check their weight gain, ensuring they are feeding well, endless diaper changes, and adjusting to life with this tiny human. It's beautiful and overwhelming all at once. And in the midst of it all, it's *so* easy to slip into the habit of complete self-neglect.

Your hormones are actually wired to keep your focus on your baby. (And let's be honest—they are incredibly adorable, so who *wouldn't* lose themselves in caring for them?) But that's exactly why this book exists—to make sure that *you,* the mother, are not forgotten.

Pelvic physical therapists and occupational therapists are dedicated to making sure you get the care you *deserve*—not just the care that has been traditionally available. We have seen firsthand how easy it is for women to be overlooked in the postpartum phase. Not because birth providers mean to neglect them, but because their job was to guide you through pregnancy and delivery. They ensured you and your baby made it through safely. But what happens next?

This is where pelvic PTs step in. Our goal is not just to help you *recover* but to help you *thrive*—to feel strong, supported, and whole in your postpartum journey.

When Should You See a Pelvic Therapist?

- If you're feeling good overall, scheduling a visit at **4-6 weeks postpartum** is ideal. This allows us to assess healing, restore core and pelvic floor function, and guide you safely back to movement.

- If you are experiencing discomfort sooner, you don't have to wait. **You can benefit from an evaluation as early as 2-3 weeks postpartum** to address immediate concerns.

What Can a Pelvic Therapist Help With?

- **Upper Back and Neck Pain:** Constant baby-holding and nursing can create tension that leads to pain and stiffness.

- **Scar Care:** Whether from a cesarean birth or perineal tears, early care can help with healing and prevent long-term tightness or discomfort.

- **Low Back or Pelvic Pain:** Pregnancy and delivery can leave behind lingering pain that needs to be addressed.

- **Orthopedic Issues:** Common postpartum conditions like *mom thumb* (De Quervain's tenosynovitis) or tailbone pain don't have to become your new normal.

- **Muscle and Fascial Tension:** Your body worked hard through pregnancy, and tension patterns can remain long after birth if not released.

- **Bladder Leaks:** Urinary incontinence is common postpartum but NOT normal. Leaking when sneezing, laughing, or exercising is a sign that your core and pelvic floor need support.

- **Pelvic Floor Heaviness:** Feeling pressure or bulging in the pelvic area as you begin standing and walking more postpartum can indicate pelvic organ prolapse, which is best addressed early.

- **Screening for Pelvic Pain Before Returning to Intimacy:** Nearly half of all new mothers experience pain with sex postpartum, but this can be resolved with the right guidance and treatment.

- **Resolving Postpartum Pelvic Pain:** Whether it's tailbone pain, perineal pain, or deep vaginal discomfort, pelvic PTs help identify and treat the root causes so you can move and live without pain.

Revisiting the 4 Pillars of Core and Pelvic Health Postpartum

Your postpartum recovery is a continuation of the work you began during pregnancy. The same assessment principles—**breath, alignment, coor-**

dination, and strength—can guide your progress as you reconnect with your core and pelvic floor.

A pelvic therapist can assess where you are now, identify areas that need attention, and help you move toward feeling great in your body again. This process is not about perfection but about *progress*—reclaiming your strength, confidence, and ability to move without pain.

Why Postpartum Pelvic Therapy is Essential

It's time to recognize that postpartum pelvic therapy is not extra credit—it is *essential*. This care sets the course for your long-term health and prevents issues that could linger for years.

For generations, women have suffered in silence, accepting postpartum symptoms like incontinence, pelvic pain, or prolapse as "just part of being a mom." But it doesn't have to be this way. With expert guidance, you can address these challenges and prevent them from becoming lifelong issues.

Pelvic health expert PTs/OTs can support *every* aspect of your physical recovery, not just your pelvic floor or core. They can:

- **Guide Fitness:** Whether you're returning to previous activities or starting fresh, we help you build a strong foundation—from breathwork to mastering squats (because motherhood means a lot of squatting!).

- **Support Running or High-Impact Activities:** Ensuring you return safely without leaks or discomfort.

- **Help With Aesthetics:** It's okay to want to address that lower belly pooch. Pelvic therapists guide you in reconnecting with your core and scaling workouts appropriately for your postpartum body.

What to Expect When Working with a Pelvic Therapist

When you work with a pelvic therapist, you can expect comprehensive, compassionate care tailored to your unique postpartum journey:

- **Comprehensive Assessment:** A full-body evaluation of your core, pelvic floor, and overall alignment, considering everything from your neck to your feet.

- **Hands-On Techniques:** Targeted care for areas like your neck, upper back, and hips, which are often strained postpartum, alongside soft tissue work for scar and muscle tension.

- **Personalized Treatment Plans:** Strategies that fit your life with a newborn, blending exercises, hands-on therapy, and lifestyle tips.

- **Education:** Clear guidance on posture, core engagement, bladder and bowel habits, and more.

- **Simple Home Exercises:** Achievable exercises that promote healing without overwhelming you.

- **Virtual Support:** Convenient online sessions when leaving home is difficult.

- **Progress Monitoring:** Regular adjustments to your care plan to reflect your recovery.

Empowering Your Postpartum Journey

The work you do with a pelvic therapist is not just about addressing symptoms—it's about *empowering* you to reclaim your body and move forward confidently.

You deserve to feel strong, supported, and ready to take on the challenges of motherhood. Postpartum pelvic therapy is the care that your mothers and grandmothers *did not* have access to—care that can transform your recovery and well-being for years to come.

You don't have to settle for "just normal." You don't have to wait until issues get worse. You don't have to accept discomfort as a lifelong consequence of childbirth.

With the right care, **you can thrive.**

Progress may be slow, but it's still progress. Celebrate every small win, for they add up to incredible change.

Chapter 42
Your Next Steps
Healing, Thriving, and Beyond

As you move forward in your postpartum recovery, remember that this journey is unique to you. There is no deadline for healing—postpartum is now considered a seven-year period, giving you the time and space to recover, rebuild, and thrive. If you're ready to take the next step, resources are available to guide you. You can find a local pelvic physical therapist at www.pelvicglobal.com or www.pelvicrehab.com, or you can work with me or my team directly, either locally or virtually, by visiting www.pinnaclewt.com.

For additional support, the **Birth Ready Bundle** is designed to equip you with tools, checklists, and resources to enhance your physical, nutritional, and mental preparation for pregnancy and postpartum. You'll find a detailed checklist of everything included at the front of this book, and I encourage you to download it as a companion to your journey.

It has been an honor to walk alongside countless women since I became a pelvic health specialist in 2010, helping them prepare for birth, recover postpartum, and reclaim their strength and confidence. My own first birth was anything but perfect, but the lessons I've learned since then have transformed my life and the lives of the women I've worked with. As one of the first pelvic PTs to integrate birth coaching, it has brought me immense joy to hear how well births have gone after working together.

This book is the culmination of all I've learned and taught, fusing the physical, nutritional, and mental aspects of this transformative time. I hope it serves you well and inspires a new standard for birthing women everywhere. You deserve to heal fully, to thrive in your motherhood journey, and to approach this chapter of your life with confidence and joy.

Rest isn't just recovery, it's rebuilding. Give yourself grace to heal.

What are ways you can be supported by others in order to rest and recover?

Your journey so far and the small wins that are building your strength.

What is one smalll step that has helped you feel more like yourself postpartum?

Healing takes time, but small, intentional actions can make a big difference.

What aspect of your recovery needs more attention or care currently?

How can your partner or support team help you during this stage of recovery?

Just as I cared for my baby during pregnancy, now is the time to care for myself. I deserve the same love and attention.

Chapter 43
Your Birth Story
Reflect and Cherish

THE POSTPARTUM PERIOD IS a time of profound transformation—a blend of emotions, new routines, and unforgettable moments. Amid the busyness, taking a moment to reflect on your birth story can feel grounding and meaningful. These pages are here whenever you're ready, whether it's a few words capturing the key moments or a detailed account of how everything unfolded. Writing your story can become a cherished keepsake—a window into one of the most powerful and transformative days of your life.

My Birth Story

What were the most memorable moments from labor and delivery?

My Birth Story

How did you feel during each stage of labor and when you first held your baby?

My Birth Story

What are you most proud of when you think
about your birth experience?

My Birth Story

What advice would you give to another mother
about the birth process?

My Birth Story

What do you want to remember about this day?

Birth Ready Resources

PREGNANCY, LABOR, POSTPARTUM AND Lactation

Our "Birth Ready" book is enriched with insights from both scientific studies and practical guides. Here's a curated list of references, each accompanied by a PMID for easy access, and a selection of foundational books that have shaped our understanding of pregnancy, childbirth, and early motherhood.

Journal Articles:

1. **Perineal Massage for Prevention of Perineal Trauma and Episiotomy During Labor:** Explores the effectiveness of perineal massage in preventing perineal trauma during childbirth. *Journal of Family Reproductive Health, Sep 2022.* PMID: 36569262.

2. **Relation between Maternal Haemoglobin Concentration and Birth Weight:** Investigates the link between a mother's haemoglobin levels and the birth weight of her baby across different ethnic groups. *BMJ, Feb 1995.* PMID: 7888886.

3. **Iron, Copper, and Fetal Development:** Discusses the roles of minerals like iron and copper in fetal development. Proceedings

of The Nutrition Society, Dec 2004. *PMID: 15831127*

4. **Minerals in Amniotic Fluid and Their Relations to Maternal and Fetal Health:** Examines the concentrations of minerals in amniotic fluid. *Biological Trace Element Research, Nov 2015. PMID: 26547910.*

5. **Role of Lysyl Oxidase Like 1 in Postpartum Connective Tissue Metabolism:** Explores the enzyme's role in postpartum connective tissue regulation. *Biology of Reproduction, Nov 2019. PMID: 31403161.*

6. **Perineal Injuries in Home Birth Settings:** A Swedish study on the impacts of home birthing practices. *BMC Pregnancy and Childbirth, Jan 2011. PMID: 21244665.*

7. **Evaluating Maternal Positions in Childbirth:** Assesses the effects of various maternal positions during childbirth. *European Journal of Midwifery, Dec 2021. PMID: 35005482.*

8. **Alternative Birthing Positions:** Compares alternative birthing positions to conventional ones during the second stage of labor. *Cureus, Apr 2023. PMID: 37223195.*

9. **Magnesium in Pregnancy:** *Nutrition Reviews, Volume 74, Issue 9, September 2016, Pages 549–557. Published: 19 July 2016.*

10. **Supplementation of Magnesium in Pregnancy:** *Spätling, et al. Journal of Pregnancy and Child Health, 4(1), 2017. DOI: 10.4172/2376-127X.1000302.*

Books:

1. *Magnesium Deficiency in the Pathogenesis of Disease:* Mildred S. Seelig, MD, MPH, FACN

2. *Real Food for Pregnancy: The Science and Wisdom of Optimal Prenatal Nutrition:* Lily Nichols, Feb 21, 2018

3. *Ina May's Guide to Childbirth:* **Updated With New Material:** Ina May Gaskin, Mar 4, 2003

4. *The Womanly Art of Breastfeeding: Completely Revised and Updated 8th Edition:* Diane Wiessinger, Diana West, Teresa Pitman, Jul 13, 2010

5. *Breastfeeding Made Simple: Seven Natural Laws for Nursing Mothers:* Nancy Mohrbacher and Kathleen Kendall-Tackett

6. *Latch: A Handbook for Breastfeeding with Confidence at Every Stage:* Robin Kaplan, M.Ed., IBCLC

7. *The Breastfeeding Atlas:* Barbara Wilson-Clay and Kay Hoover

8. *The Birth Partner:* Penny Simkin — An essential guide for partners, doulas, and other support people involved in the birth process.

9. *Reclaiming Childbirth as a Rite of Passage: Weaving Ancient Wisdom with Modern Knowledge:* Rachel Reed — This book integrates ancient wisdom with modern practices to provide

a holistic view of the birth experience.

10. ***Mayo Clinic Guide to a Healthy Pregnancy:*** Mayo Clinic Staff — A comprehensive guide offering week-by-week insights and advice for expecting parents.

These resources serve as a foundation for understanding the complex and beautiful journey of pregnancy and childbirth. Each piece of literature, whether a research article or a book, contributes to a holistic view of maternal health and well-being.

About the Author

In *Birth Ready and Beyond*, author and pelvic physical therapist **Buffy Stinchfield** draws from over sixteen years of experience helping women feel strong, capable, and confident through every stage of pregnancy and postpartum recovery.

Inspired by both her personal journey and her professional practice, Stinchfield wrote this book to honor her past self—and to empower other women with the knowledge, preparation, and compassion they deserve.

Too often, pre and postnatal care focuses solely on the baby, leaving mothers without the physical, emotional, and functional support they need.

Birth Ready and Beyond was created to change that narrative. Combining evidence-based physical therapy with heart-centered guidance, the book offers an integrated approach to self-care before, during, and after birth.

Designed as both an educational guide and an interactive workbook, it includes narrative insight, at-home physical therapy exercises, self-assessments, journaling prompts, nourishing recipes, and more. Each section is easy to navigate, allowing readers to find what they need—when they need it.